# MIXED MARTIAL ARTS (MMA) STRIKERS GUIDE
## for TRAINERS and FIGHTERS

By; Joseph Paulo Florez de la Guevara
aka: Joe Guevara

*AuthorHouse™*
*1663 Liberty Drive*
*Bloomington, IN 47403*
*www.authorhouse.com*
*Phone: 1-800-839-8640*

*First published by AuthorHouse 3/16/2010*

*ISBN: 978-1-4490-9612-0 (sc)*

*Library of Congress Control Number: 2010903404*

*Printed in the United States of America*
*Bloomington, Indiana*

*This book is printed on acid-free paper.*

# SPECIAL THANKS

A special thanks to my Dad who instilled in me the training ethics I hold so dear to my heart. For without them, I would not have be able to succeed in my personal training, my training other's throughout the years, and being able to manage and train over his Capitol Boxing Gym when he got ill and eventually passed.

To Jerome "Jerry" Jacobs, my mentor and friend in boxing, Jerry made me a better man and boxer. He took a scrappy young kid and made him a force to be reckoned with in the boxing world, both as an amateur and a professional.

To Amy Williams my friend and to whom I am grateful for pushing me into the MMA field instead of working at other venues.

My utmost appreciation goes to the men and women, boys and girls that I've trained at the Capitol Boxing Gymnasium and the Ultimate Fitness Training Center in Sacramento, California.

Special thanks go out to Uriah Faber and Matt Fisher for allowing me to sharpen my skills at their Ultimate Fitness Mixed Martial Arts Training Center in Sacramento. They were very instrumental in forcing me to write this guide book and sharing my knowledge of the sport.

I will always be grateful…

My greatest thanks goes to My God, for giving me the strength; mentally, physically, and spiritually to fulfill my path in life with love, honor, respect, pride, and courage. In all that I've accomplished both in and out of the ring.

Joseph Paulo Florez. de la Guevara aka: Joe Guevara

| **Photo models:** | **Photographers:** | **Audits:** |
|---|---|---|
| Ignacio Anguiano | KT Jorgenson | Dr. Saralyn Bregman |
| Saralyn Bregman | Mark Renteria | |
| Danny Castillo | | |
| Stephanie Corbitt | **Assistant:** | **Composition:** |
| Kristana Erikson | Catherine Espinoza | Wayne Cain |
| Jeremy Freitag | | |
| Erin Gallegos | | |
| Rick Inzunza | | |
| Joe Nelson | | |
| Emmett Smith | | |
| Mario Soto | | |
| Other guy behind counter... | | |

# TABLE OF CONTENTS

# VII SPARRING, FIGHT DAY, & CONCLUSION

## Sparring

### Fight day

# LIST OF ILLUSTRATIONS

## VI BAG DRILLS

## VII SPARRING, FIGHT DAY, & CONCLUSION

# MIXED MARTIAL ARTS (MMA) STRIKERS GUIDE
# FOR TRAINERS AND FIGHTERS

By Joseph Paulo Florez de la Guevara aka: Joe Guevara
January 9, 2009

## INTRODUCTION

The primary motive in Boxing and Mixed Martial Arts (MMA) Striking (herein called Striking) is to deliver a blow to some part of an opponent's anatomy while at the same time avoiding a counter. The quicker the blow, the more disconcerting it will be for your opponent and the better you will be able to recover yourself for another attack.

Throughout the years there have been many boxers, and as of lately many, MMA Fighting Champions who have a special piece about them that distinguishes them from other fighters. This book helps to identify some of those differences.

Boxer's can only punch with two things, their fists. The MMA Fighter can strike with eights things; both of their hands, elbows, knees, and feet. What will be addressed in this book is mainly hand and elbow strikes.

There are at least 7-Jabs of Champions, four-defenses, and various positions for both offensive and defensive attacks. The Bull-Dog Defense (Stalking) is the best as it forces the pace and enables the fighter to obtain the best offensive position on an opponent.

There is a correct way to Shadow-Box using power and control. With this one exercise a boxer can develop his strength, stamina, control, defense, positioning, and combinations. The mirror exercise is a valuable tool to use with shadow boxing. When used correctly, a fighter is able to practice his defensive combinations, counter punching skills, knowledge of where to hit, gain control of his punches, and work on his footwork. Using these exercises, one can build on the shadow-boxing skills and subsequently their defensive and offensive combinations. These and more exercises are described below for your viewing pleasure.

## I. FIST/HANDWRAPS

### Fist

- **How to make a Fist:**

  Every fighter should practice the right method of doubling the fist and knowing how to hit with the knuckles. This will aid the fighter in avoiding dislocated joints and broken bones. When closing the fist, bring the tips of the fingers well over and tucked into the palm. The thumb is turned inside and over the first joint of the index and middle fingers. See figure CI-01

- **Basic hitting:**

  Basic hitting utilizes all four knuckles. Basic hitting consists of jabs, fast combinations, and set up punches. See figure CI-02

- **Hard hitting:**

  Hard hitting utilizes the two knuckles of the index and middle fingers. Hard damaging punches are aimed at specific soft (weak) spots of the head and body. See figures CI-03, CI-A & CI-B

## Hand Wrap Guide

- **Types and Sizes of Handwraps**

  There are many types of handwraps which can be broken down by size. There is the **cotton herringbone** or the **elastic**, 2"x 120" up to 2"x 180", for training. The US Amateur Boxing rules refer to them as **velpeau (training wraps).** The **gauze**, 2"x 10 yards up to 2"x 15 yards, is used for competition. See figure CI-04

  The **cotton herringbone** does not stretch, are reusable, and should be washed after each use. The **elastic** style, better known as the Mexican Handwraps (because they are often made in Mexico), have some stretch to them and tend to be more comfortable. They are also reusable and should be washed after each use.

  The **gauze** (soft surgical bandage) hand wrap is mostly used in amateur and professional competition and used by some professionals during training. They are not used much in gymnasiums since they are disposable and therefore not the most practical. Gauze has no give, is much thinner, and is used with **trainers** tape (surgeon's adhesive tape).

- **Functions**

  Wrapping ones hands for the **gymnasium** is subject to preference of type, style, and size of hand wrap. The main thing to remember is that the purpose of the wrap is to protect the hand from injury.

  Protection from injury also applies to the **amateur and professional competition** wraps except that they are guided legally by the California State Athletic Commission's (CSAC) Rules; and are inspected and cleared by the CSAC's trained Athletic Inspectors' prior to competition.

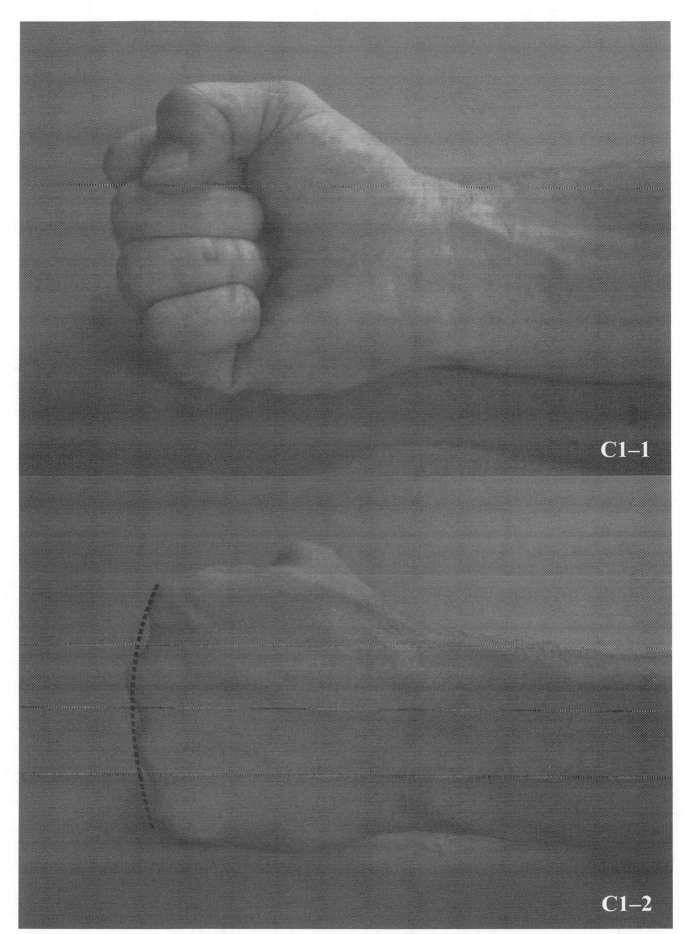

C1–1

C1–2

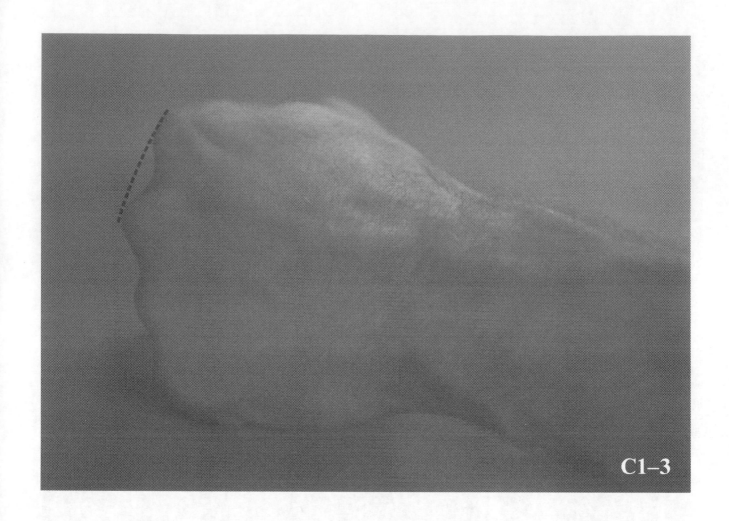

C1–3

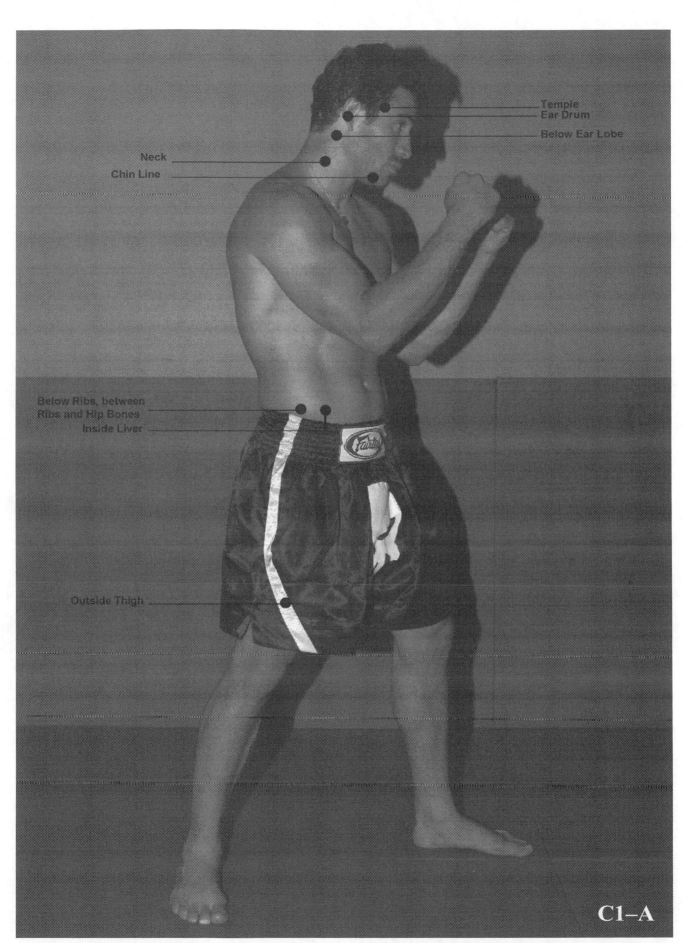

Temple
Ear Drum
Below Ear Lobe
Neck
Chin Line
Below Ribs, between
Ribs and Hip Bones
Inside Liver
Outside Thigh

C1–A

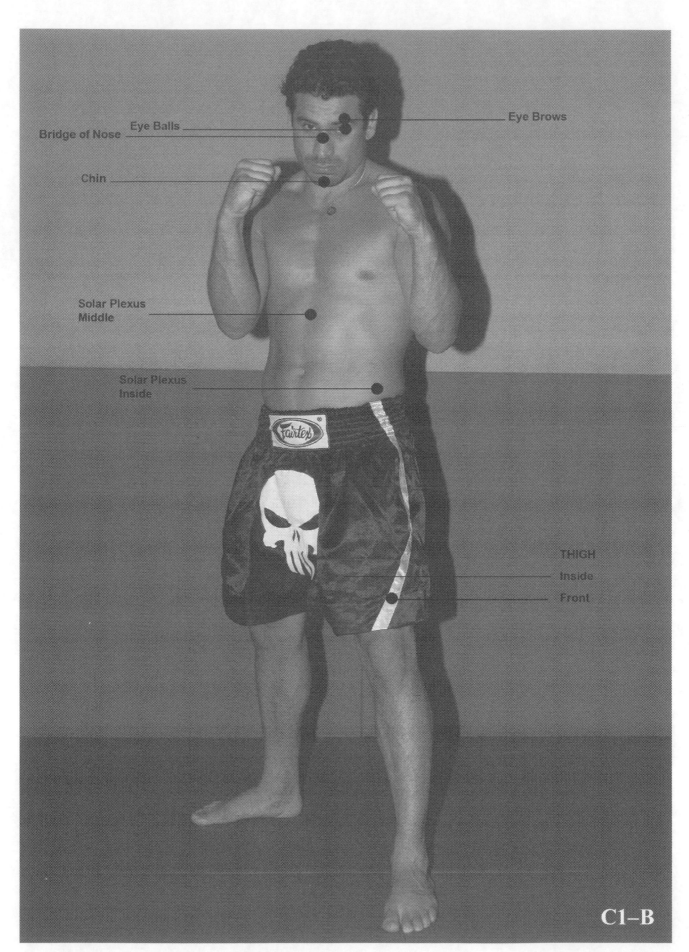

Bridge of Nose

Eye Balls

Eye Brows

Chin

Solar Plexus
Middle

Solar Plexus
Inside

THIGH

Inside

Front

**C1–B**

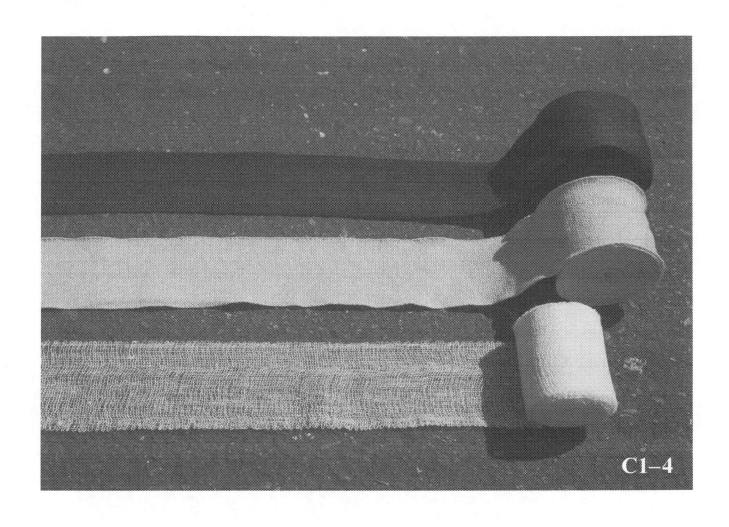

C1–4

# NOTES

## Style of Wraps for Training Purposes

The **Basic** handwrap is for beginners or younger fighters. This wrap does not go between the fingers as the hands may not yet be developed and may be too small.

- Start with the palm facing down, with fingers spread apart. Keep the hand spread at all times while wrapping. This insures that when you make a fist and your hand expands the wrap, it will feel firm but not tight. Loop the hand wrap over the thumb. Next pull away from thumb and wrap around the wrist a few times. See figures CI-05 & CI-06

- Proceed to wrap around the knuckles a few times. A rule of thumb is to match the edge of the wrap with the middle knuckles of the fingers; this way when you make a fist the wrap will cover all the knuckles. Check for firmness. See figures CI-07 & CI-08

- Come back up, wrap completely around the thumb, and check for firmness. See figures CI-09 & CI-10

- Go back to the wrist, then to the knuckles, and then to the back of the hand, keeping the wraps neat and evenly distributed. Check firmness. See figures CI-11 & CI-12

- Finish up at the wrist. See figures CI-13 & CI-14

The **Advanced I (Untucked)** is one of the more widely used methods of wrapping for both the amateur and professional fighter. It wraps between the fingers but is not tucked under the palm.

- Starting with the palm facing down and fingers spread apart. Keep the hand spread at all times while wrapping. This way, when you make a fist and your hand expands the wrap will feel firm and not tight. Loop the hand wrap over the thumb, pull away from the thumb, and wrap around wrist a few times. See figures CI-15 & CI-16

- Next proceed to wrap around the knuckles a few times. A rule of thumb is to match the edge of the wrap with the middle knuckles of the fingers. This way when you make a fist the wrap will cover all the knuckles. Check for firmness. See figures CI-17 & CI-18

- Wrap completely around the thumb and check for firmness. See figures CI-19 & CI-20

- Bring the wraps between the fingers starting at the outside or inside finger coming over the thumb each time and check for firmness. See figures CI-21 thru 22

- Bring the wrap back under the palm and around the knuckles to clean it up. Finish up at the wrist. See figures CI-23, CH-24, & CI-25

The **Advanced II (Tucked)** is one of the lesser used methods of wrapping for both the amateur and professional fighter. It wraps between the fingers but is also tucked under the palm. Some will like the added grip it gives with the added wrap on the palm while others will not.

- Start with the palm facing down and fingers spread apart. Keep the hand spread at all times while wrapping. This way when you make a fist and your hand expands the wrap will feel firm and not tight. Loop hand wraps over the thumb, pull away from the thumb and wrap around the wrist a few times. See figures CI-26 & CI-27

- Proceed to wrap around the knuckles a few times. A rule of thumb is to match the edge of the wrap with the middle knuckles of the fingers. This way, when you make a fist, the wrap will cover all the knuckles. Check for firmness. See figures CI-28 & CI-29

- Wrap completely around the thumb and check for firmness. See figures CI-30 & CI-31

- Bring the wraps between the fingers starting at the outside or inside finger coming over the thumb each time and check for firmness. See figures CI-32 thru 34

- Turn palm up and tuck the wrap into and through the wrap under the knuckles. Pull and wrap back over the thumb then back under into, and through the wrap under the knuckles. Repeat for the remaining knuckles and check for firmness. See figures CI-35 thru 37

- Bring the wrap back over hand and around the knuckles to clean it up. Finish up at the wrist. See figures CI-38 thru 41

The **Ribbon/Stack Advanced I or II** is another style that has its followers and will benefit the fighter that needs and/or wants the added cushion over the knuckles. This style is mostly used with the gauze and tape during competition and can be used with either the Advanced I or II styles above.

- Start with the palm facing down, and fingers spread apart. Keep the hand spread at all times while wrapping. This way when you make a fist and your hand expands the wrap will feel firm and not tight. Loop hand wrap over the thumb, then pull away from the thumb and wrap around the wrist a few times. See figures CI-42 & CI-43

- Next proceed to wrap around the knuckles a few times. A rule of thumb is to match the edge of the wrap with the middle knuckles of the fingers. This way when you make a fist, the wrap will cover all the knuckles. Check for firmness. See figures CI-44 & CI-45

- Now lay the wraps back and forth over the knuckles, making a ribbon or stack pattern. Hold inside edge with thumb. See figures CI-46 & CI-47

- Completely wrap around knuckles and back to wrist. See figures CI-48

- Wrap completely around the thumb. See figure CI-49

- Bring the wraps between the fingers starting at the outside or inside finger, coming over the thumb each time and check for firmness. See figures CI-50 thru 52

- Bring the wrap back under the palm and around the knuckles to clean it up. Finish up at the wrist. See figures CI-53 & CI-54

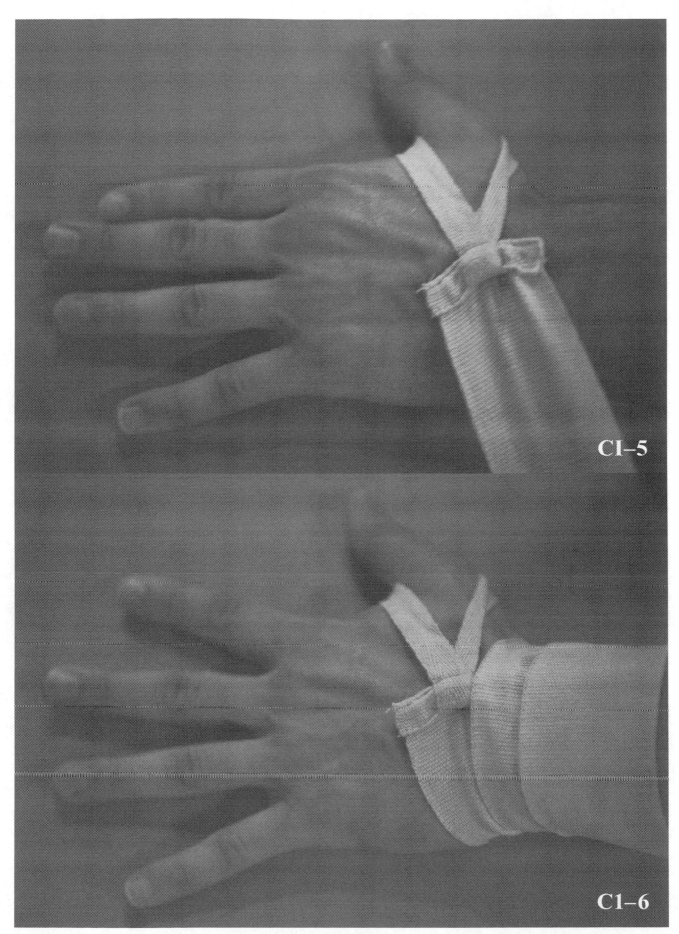

C1–5

C1–6

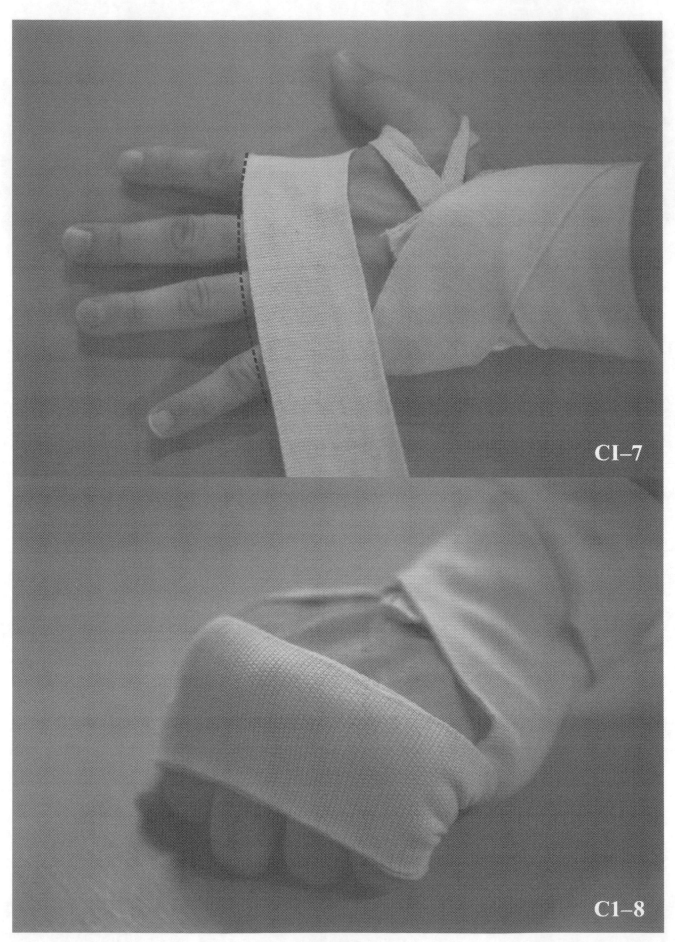

CI–7

C1–8

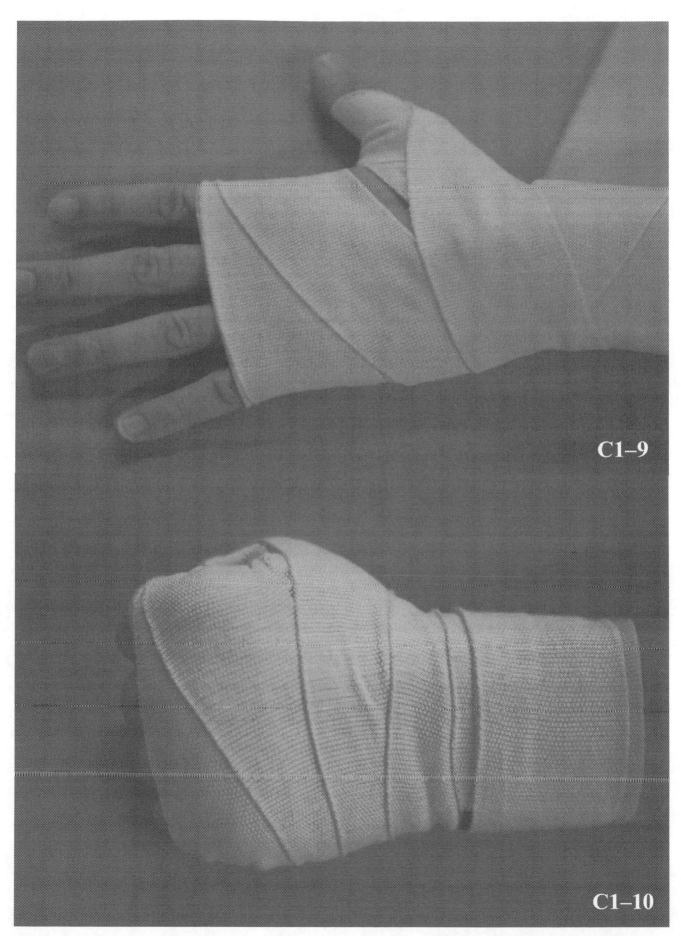

C1–9

C1–10

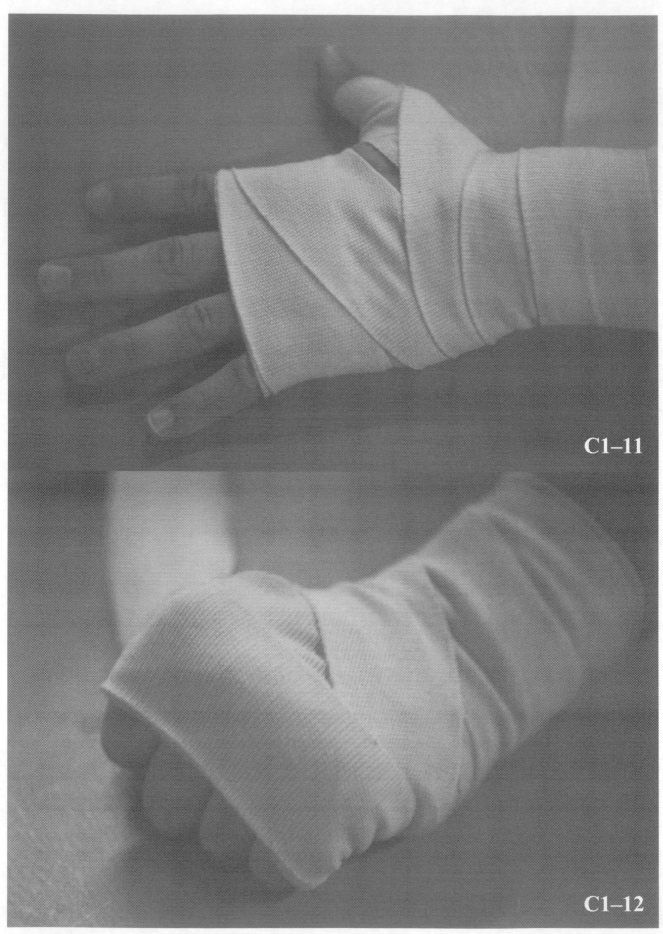

C1–11

C1–12

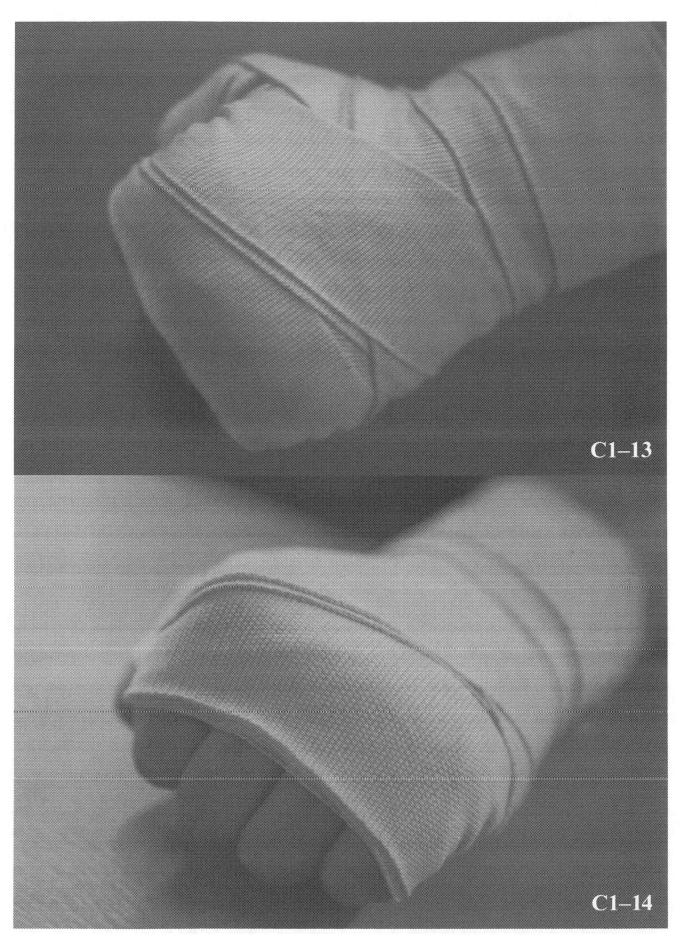

C1–13

C1–14

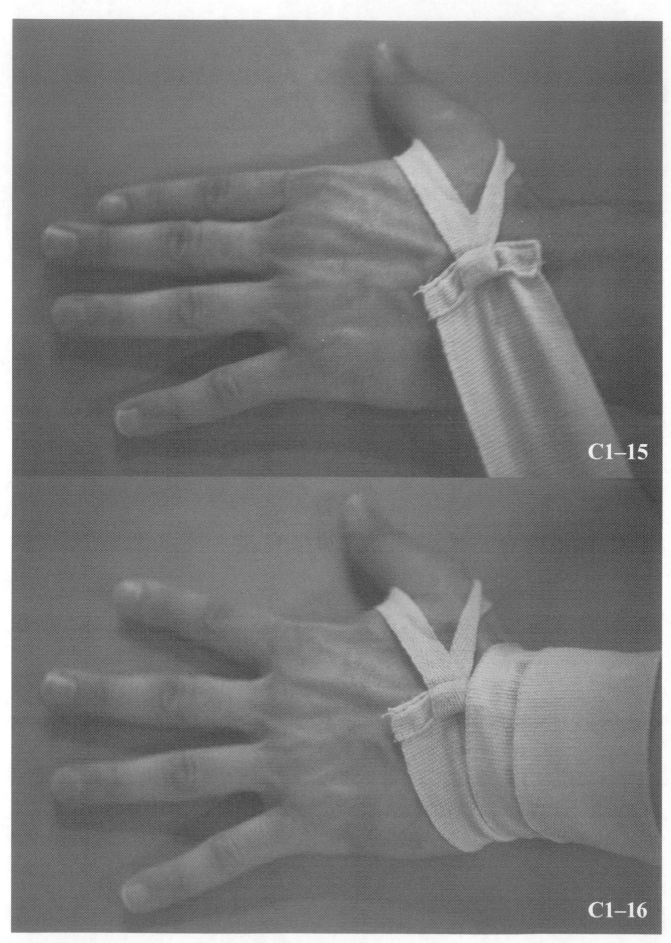

C1–15

C1–16

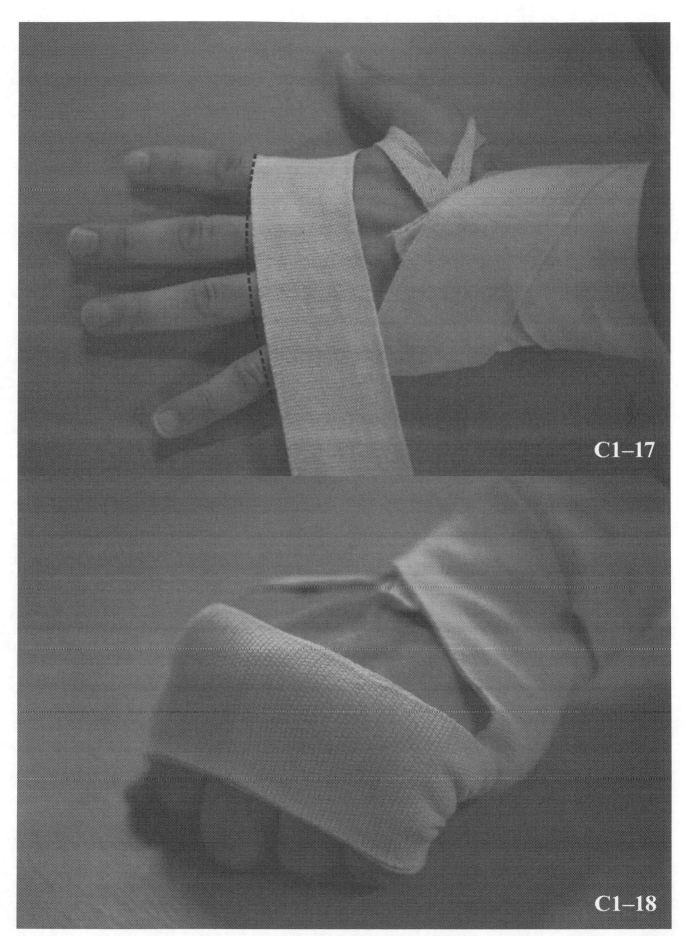

C1–17

C1–18

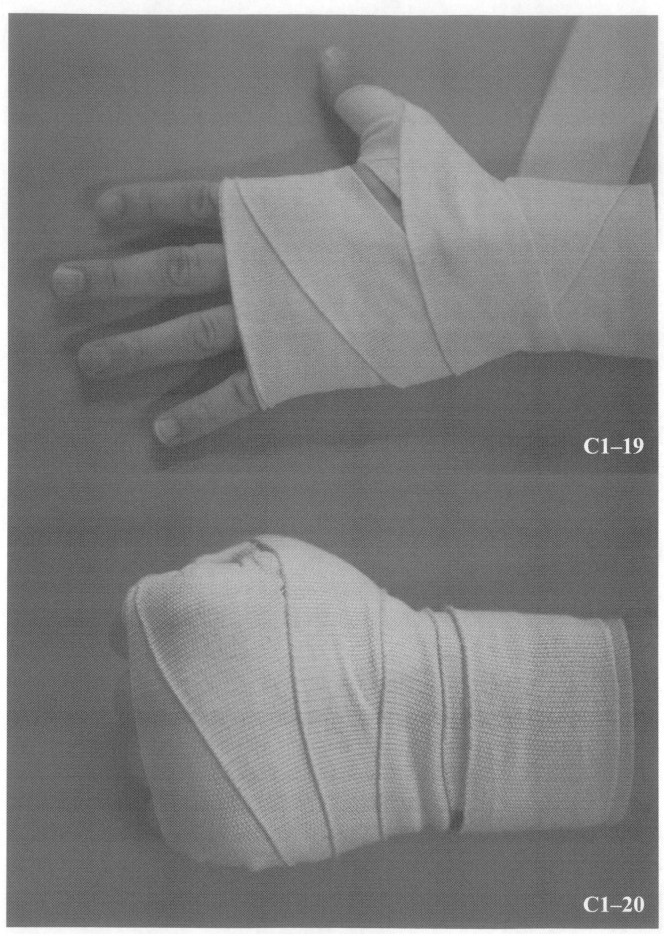

C1–19

C1–20

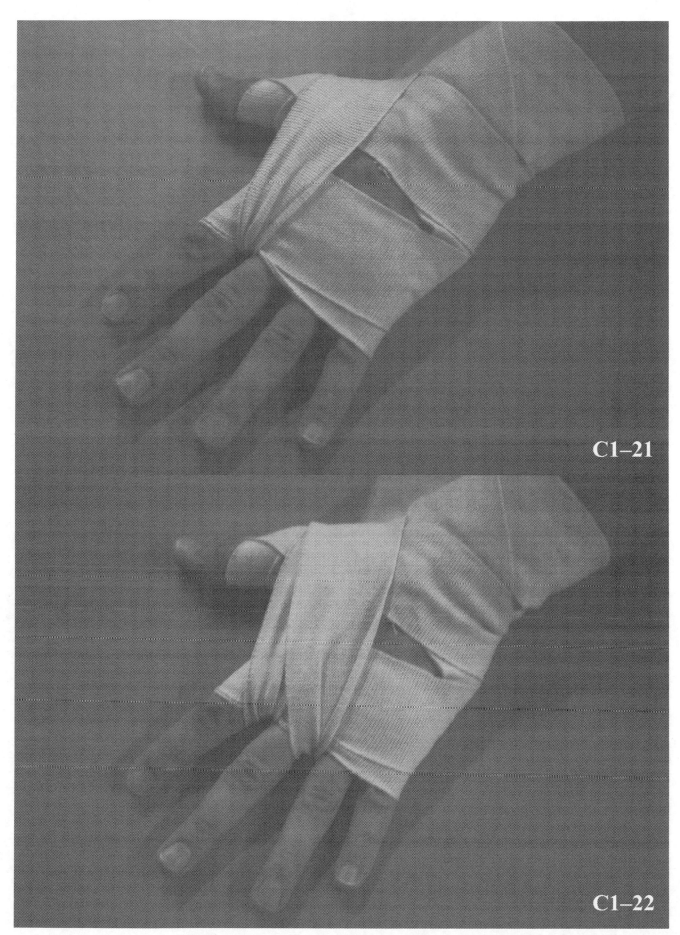

C1–21

C1–22

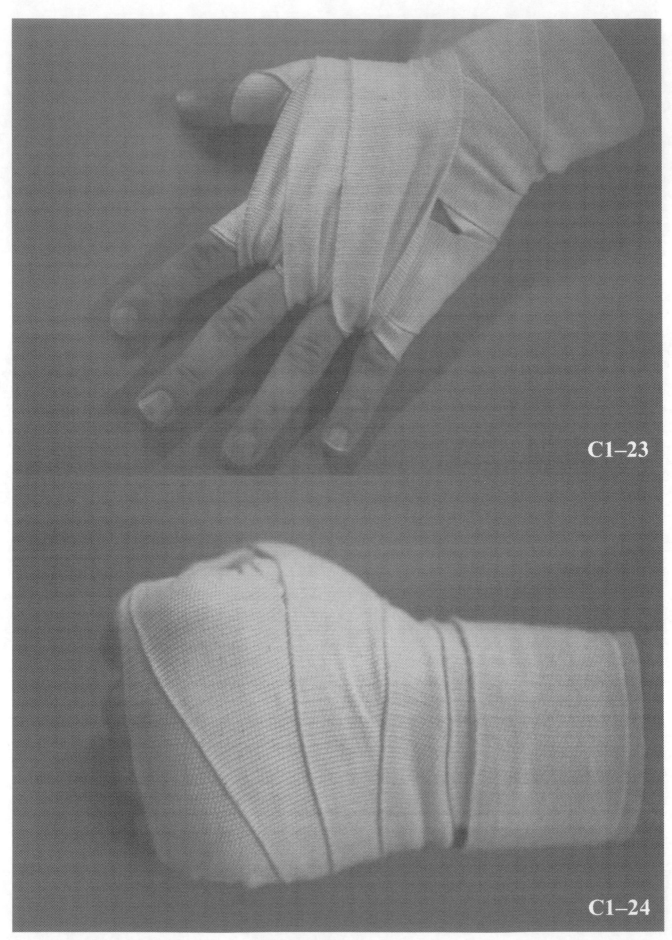

C1–23

C1–24

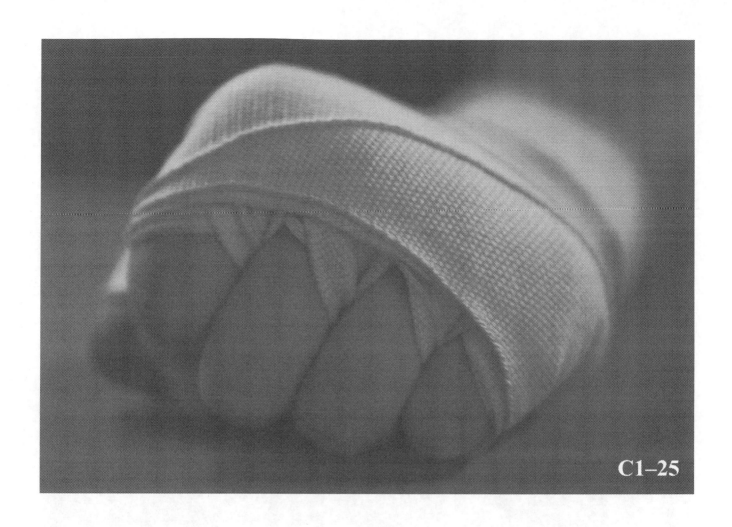

C1–25

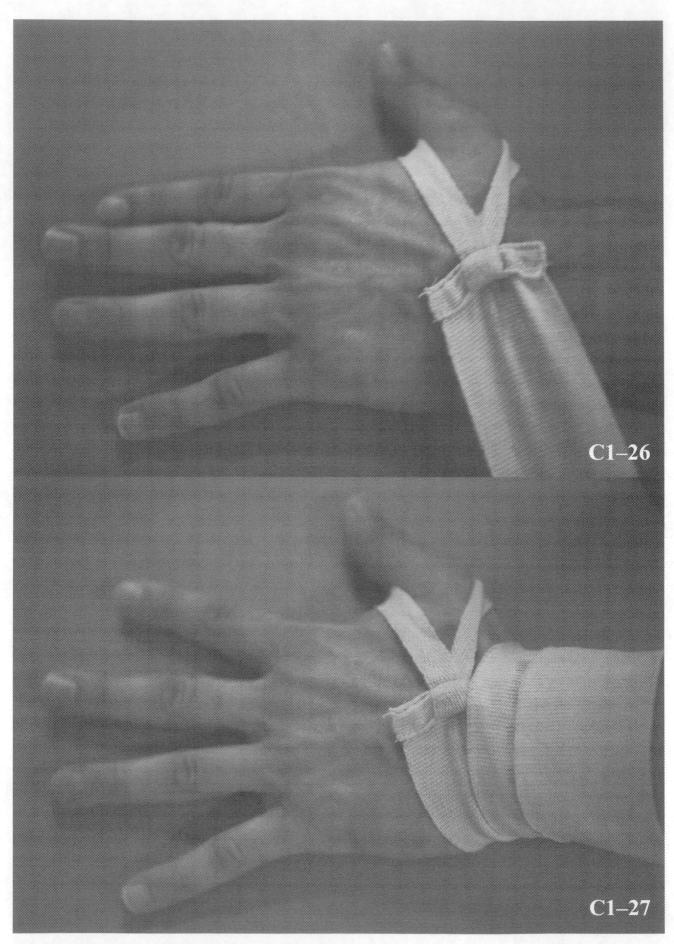

C1–26

C1–27

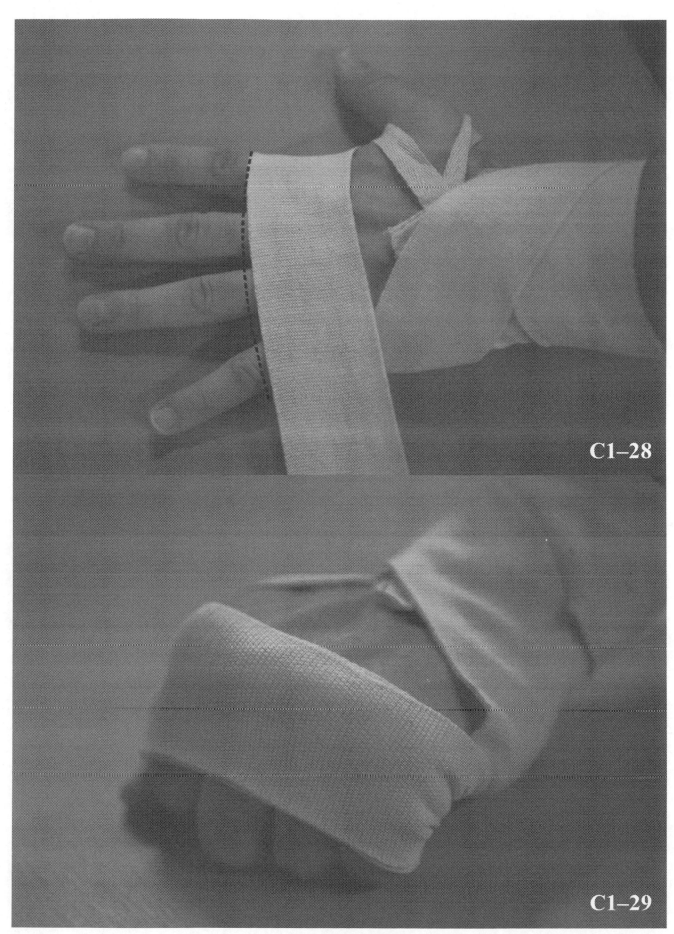

C1–28

C1–29

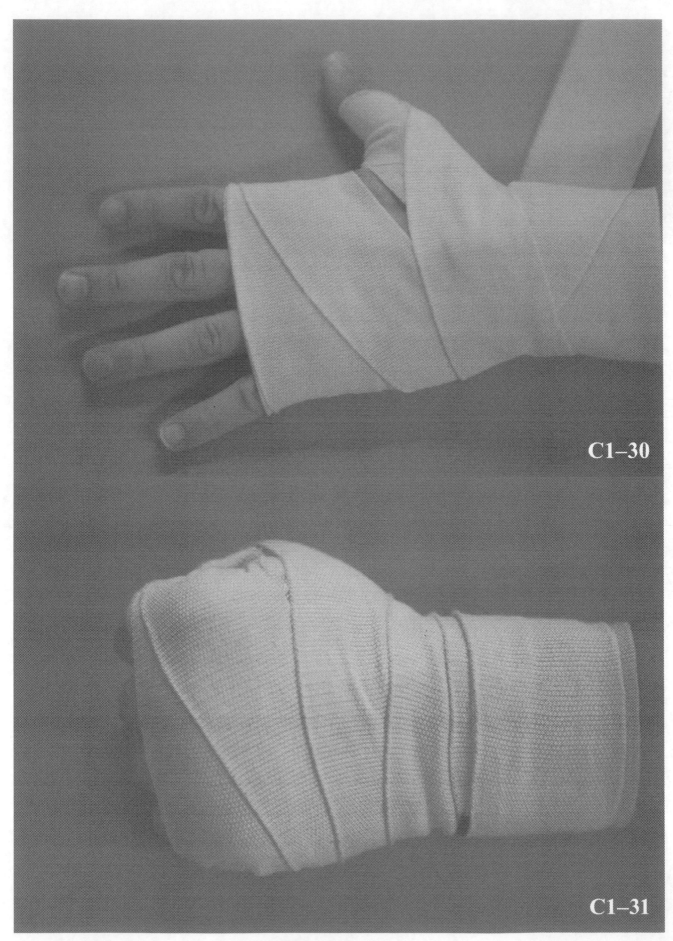

C1–30

C1–31

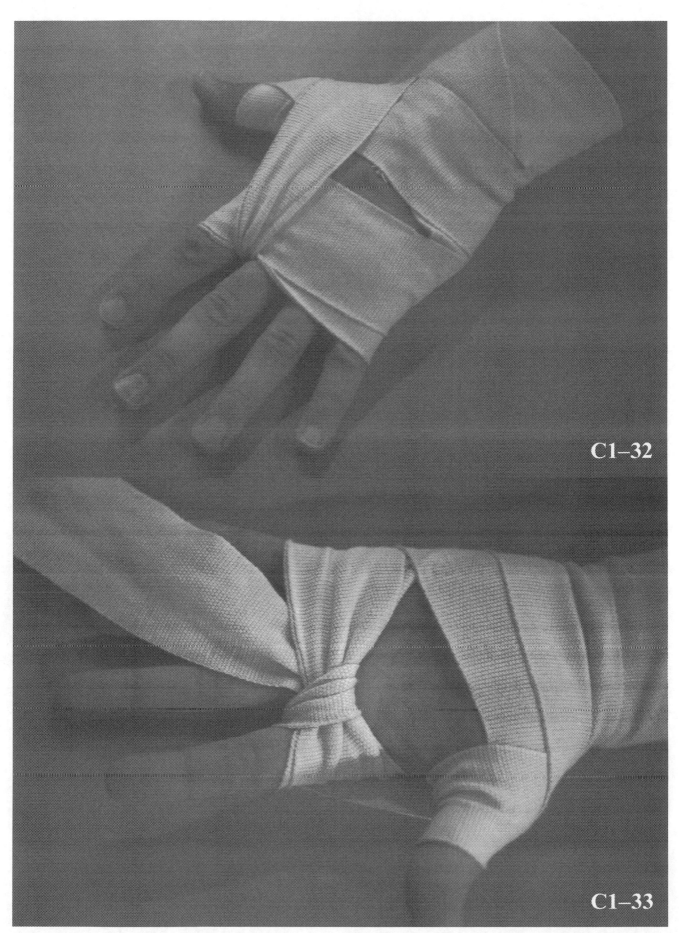

C1–32

C1–33

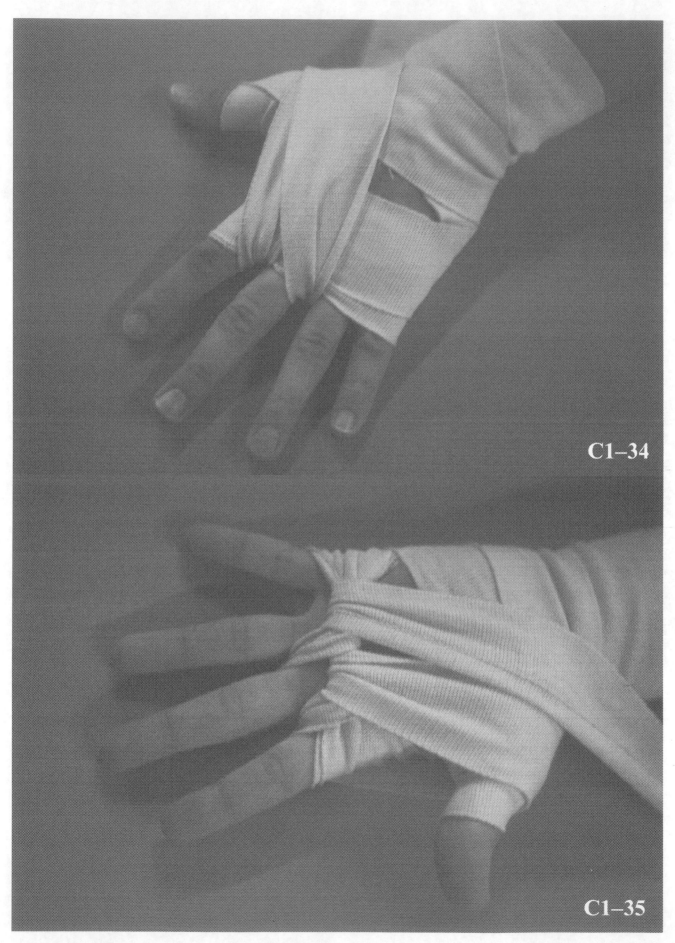

C1–34

C1–35

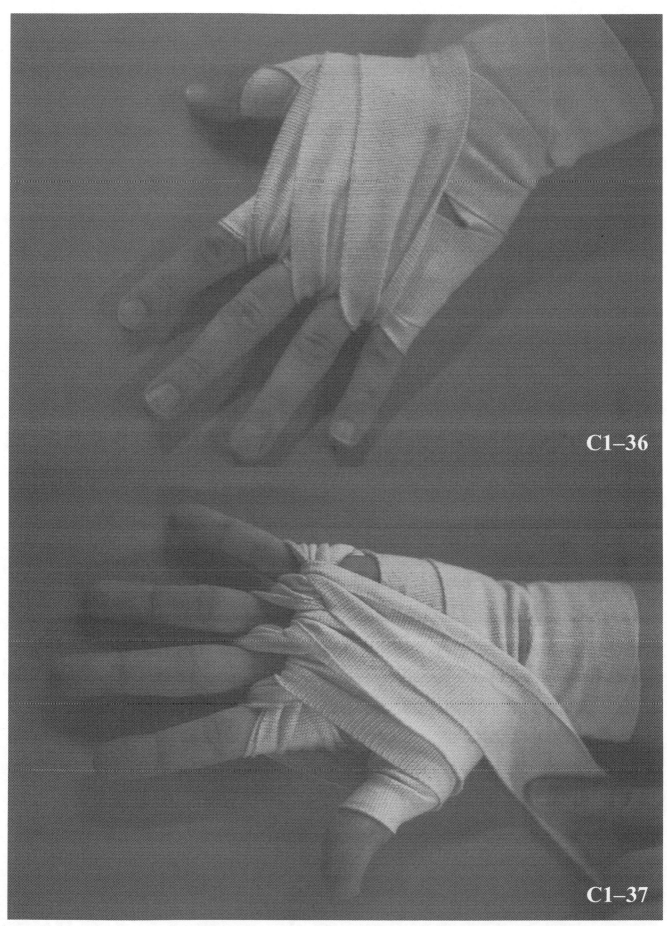

C1–36

C1–37

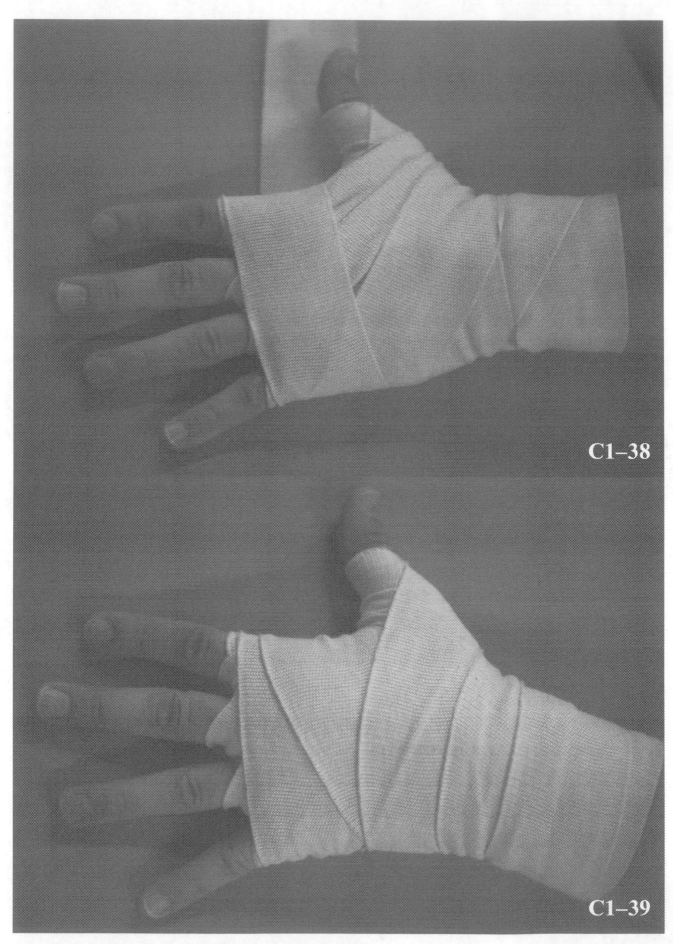

C1–38

C1–39

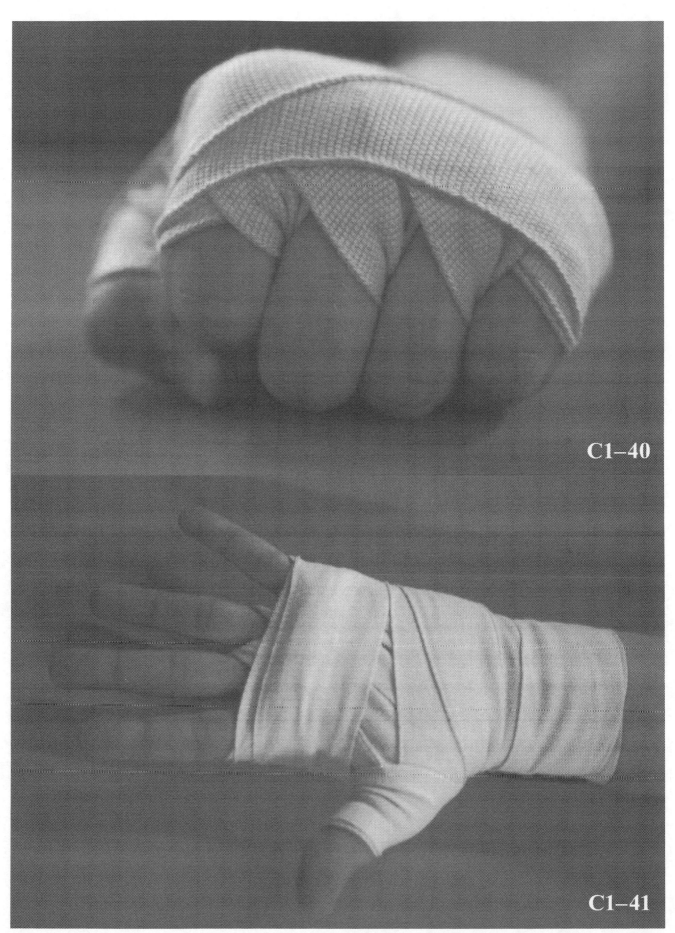

C1–40

C1–41

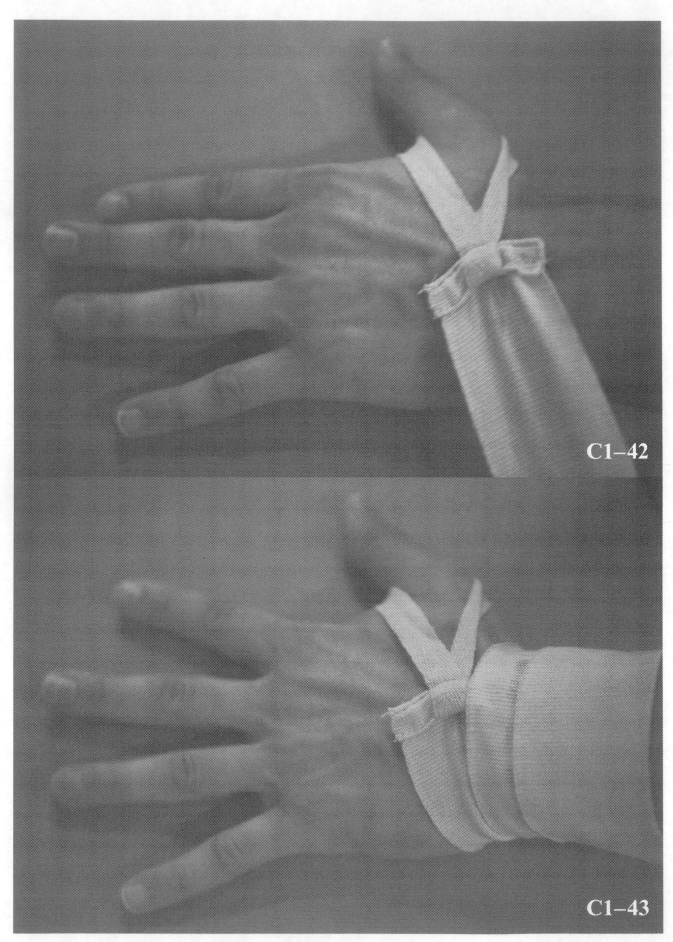

C1–42

C1–43

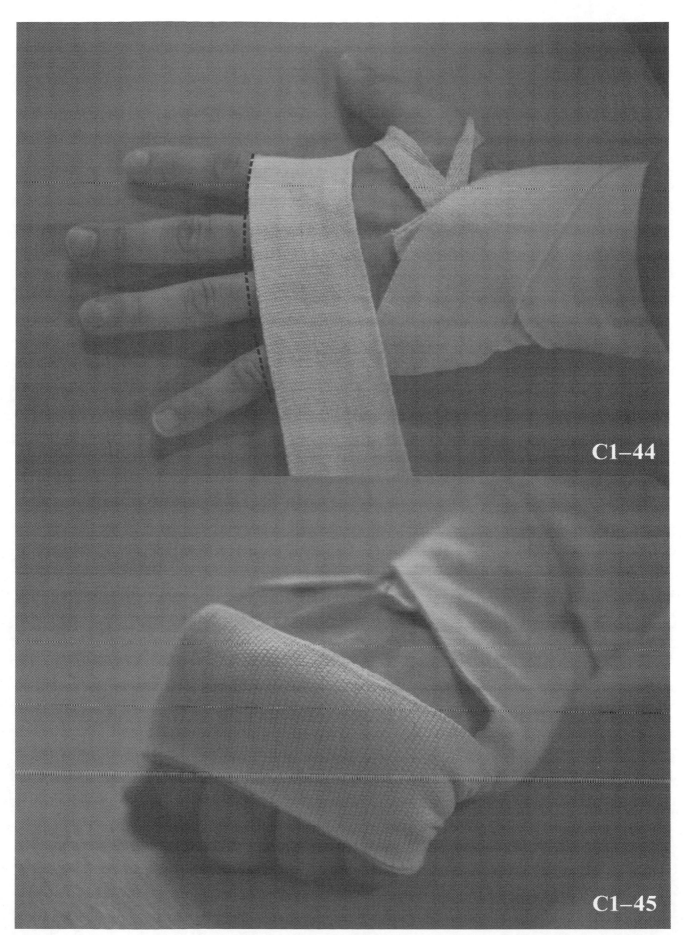

C1–44

C1–45

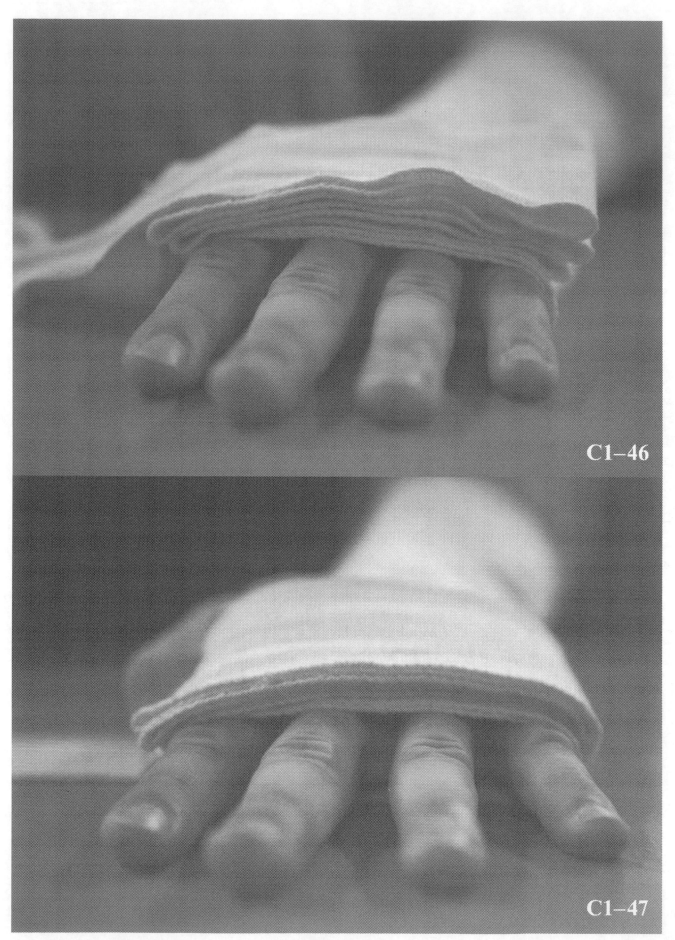

C1–46

C1–47

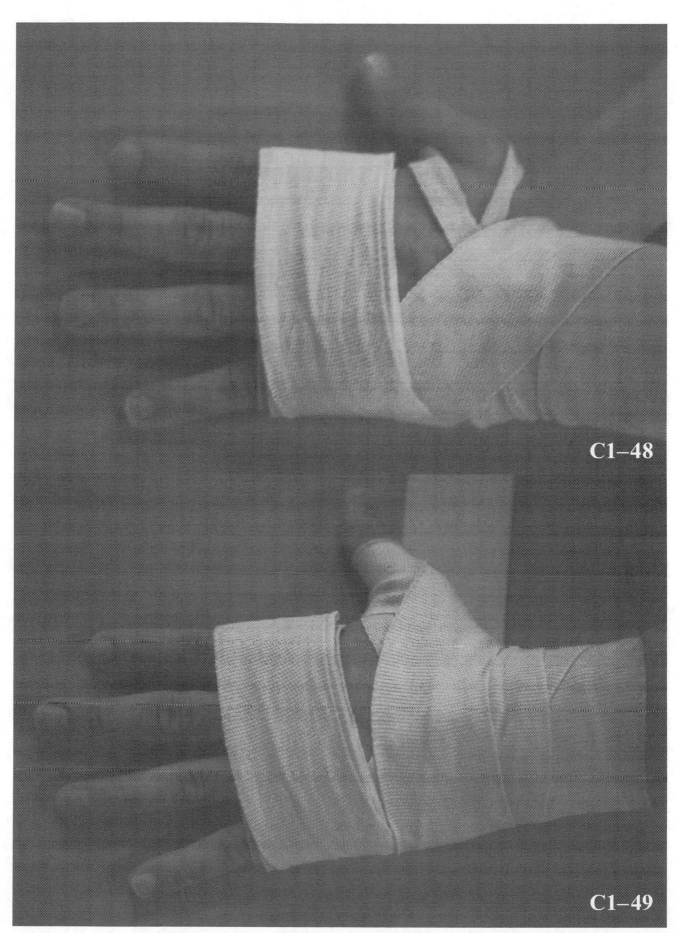

C1–48

C1–49

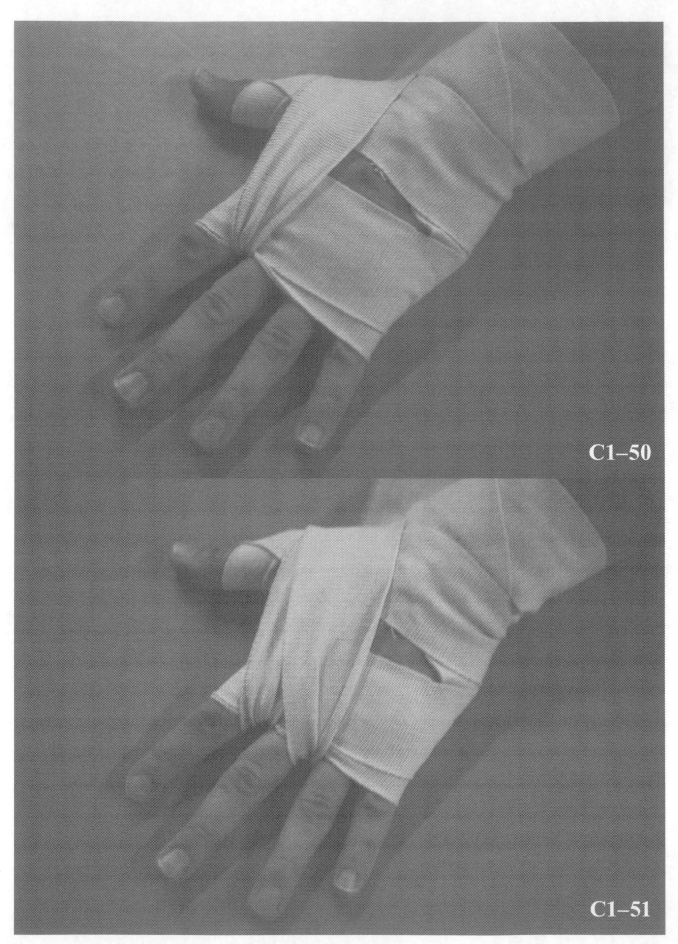

C1–50

C1–51

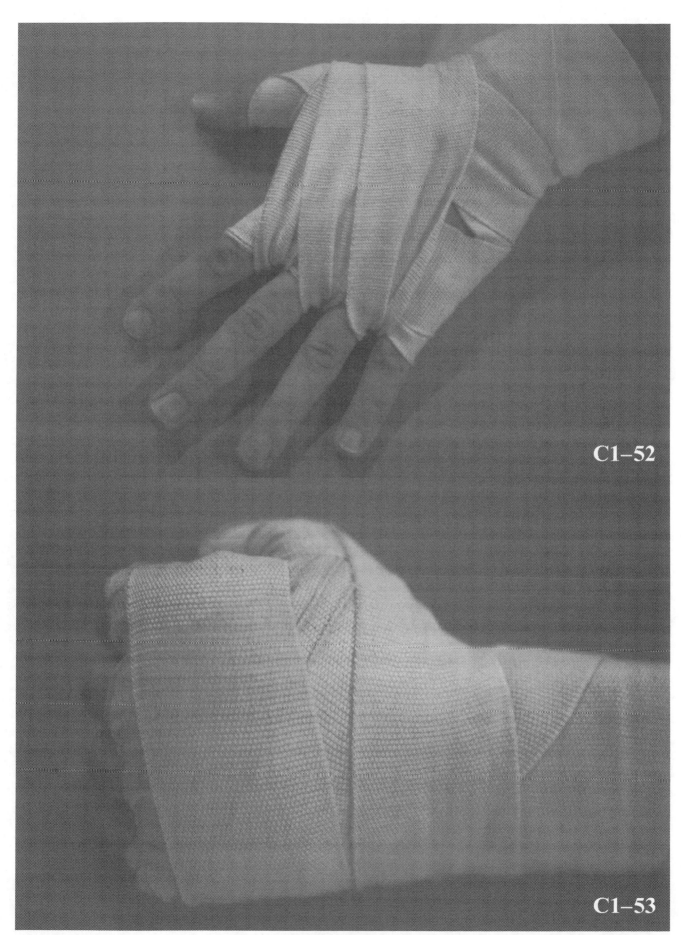

C1–52

C1–53

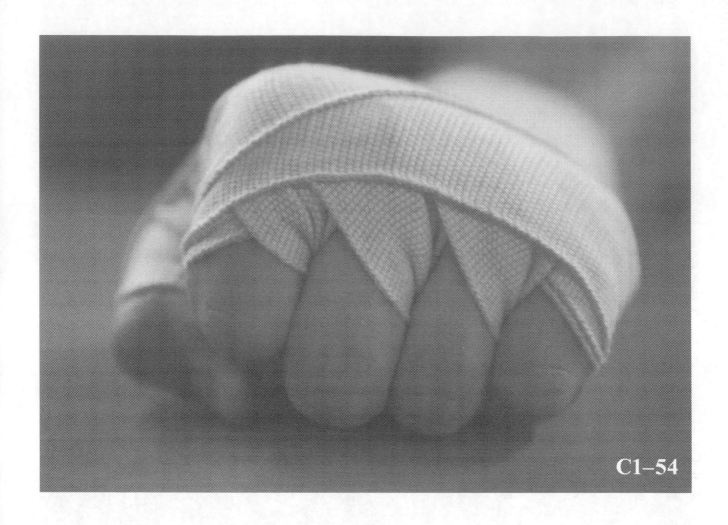

C1–54

**California State Athletic Commission (CSAC) Legal Guidelines for Amateur and Professional Competition Wraps**

- **Amateur Boxing References and Rules**

### Legal Competition Wraps for Amateur Boxers

Licensed Amateur Boxers have the option of any of the Advanced I or II styles or the Ribbon/Stack A-I or A-II styles mentioned above. Most utilize the Ribbon/Stack styles and can only use **Soft Surgical Bandage (Gauze), Surgeon's Adhesive Tape (Tape), or Velpeau (training wraps)** See figure CI-55

**All Licensed Amateur Boxers will adhere to the State Athletic Commissions Policy's listed from the United States Amateur Boxing Regulation's:**

Section 7. Bandages (USABR-Section 103.5 Bandages (handwraps) and Tape specifications)

**Surgeon's adhesive tape (tape)** over the knuckles is prohibited.

For competitions in the United States, each boxer shall wear handwraps. The use of water or any liquid or material on any part of the handwrap is strictly prohibited. Only **soft surgical bandages (gauze), surgeon's adhesive tape (tape), or velpeau (training wraps)** are allowed. See figure CI-55

Bandages should be supervised by an official specifically assigned for this purpose. The wraps should also be re-inspected before the gloves are fitted and taped for competition.

Bandages shall not exceed the following restrictions:

Amateur boxers can use (15) fifteen yards of (2") two inch **gauze** and a minimum of (3') three feet up to a maximum of (6') six feet of (1") one inch **tape** per hand. The **tape** must be applied (1") one inch behind the knuckles. Strips of **tape** placed between the fingers in the joint to hold down the bandages are permitted, but will not extend past or on the knuckles. **Tape** (1") one inch by (8") eight inches may secure the bandages around the wrist. See figures CI-56 thru CI-58

Amateur boxers can use (8') eight feet (2 ¼ ") two and one quarter inches of **Velpeau** and a minimum of (3') three feet up to a maximum of (6') six feet of (1") one inch **tape** per hand. Strips of **tape** placed between the fingers in the joint to hold down the bandages are permitted, but will not extend past or on the knuckles. **Tape** (1") one inch by (8") eight inches may secure the bandages around the wrist.
See figure CI-59

- **Amateur and Professional Kickboxing References and Rules**

### Legal Competition Wraps for Amateur and Professional Kickboxers

Licensed Amateur and Professional Kickboxers have the option of any of the Advanced I or II styles or the Ribbon/Stack A-I or A-II styles mentioned above. Most utilize the Ribbon/Stack styles and can only use **Soft Surgical Bandage (Gauze), Surgeon's Adhesive Tape (Tape), Velpeau (training wraps)** See figures CI-60

All Licensed Amateur Boxers will adhere to the State Athletic Commissions Policy's listed from the Commissions:

### "Amateur and Professional Kickboxing Rules and Referee Guidelines" 2008.

### Section 9. Bandages

Bandages are optional.

Tape over the knuckles is prohibited.

If bandages are used, don't start handwrapping without an Inspector present.

Bandages shall not exceed the following restrictions:

The use of water or any liquid or material on any part of the handwrap is strictly prohibited.

Bandages will be adjusted in the dressing room in the presence of both contestants and a Commission Representative. All bandages/wrappings are to be signed off by a Commission Representative. Either contestant may waive his privilege of witnessing the bandaging/wrapping of his opponent's hands.

Bandages will not exceed the following restrictions:

One winding of **surgeon's adhesive tape**, not over one and one-half inches wide, placed directly on the hand to protect that part of the hand near the wrist. Said tape may cross the back of the hand twice but will not extend within one-inch of the knuckles when the hand is clenched to make a fist. See figure CI-61

Contestants will use **soft surgical bandage**, not over two inches wide, held in place by no more than eight (8) feet of **surgeon's adhesive tape** for each hand. One thirty (30) yard roll of **bandage** should complete the wrapping for each hand.
See figures CI-62 thru CI-66

- **Professional Boxer References and Rules**

### Professional Boxer

Licensed Professional Boxers have the option of any of the Advanced I or II styles or the Ribbon/Stack style mentioned above. Most utilize the Ribbon/Stack styles and can only use Soft Surgical Bandage **(Gauze)** and Surgeon's Adhesive Tape **(Tape)**. See figure CI-67

**All Professional Boxers will adhere to the State Athletic Commissions Policy's listed from the Commissions:**

**"Professional Boxing Rules" 2009.**
**Bandages and Handwraps**

Advise the Chief Second that the wrapping and gloving of the participant must be done in the presence of an Inspector. If a wrap has started without supervision, kindly ask to have the wrap removed and restarted in the presence of an Inspector.

In all weight classes, all bandages and hand wraps applied to each hand are restricted to:

**Section 323. Bandages**
Bandages shall not exceed the following restrictions:

One winding of **surgeon's adhesive tape**, not over one and one-half inches wide, placed directly on the hand to protect that part of the hand near the wrist. Said tape may cross the back of the hand twice but shall not extend within one inch of the knuckles when hand is clenched to make a fist. See figure CI-68

Contestants shall use **soft surgical bandage** not over two inches wide, held in place by not more than ten yards of **surgeon's adhesive tape** for each hand. Not more than twenty yards of **bandage** may be used to complete the wrapping for each hand. See figures CI-69 thru CI-72

Bandages shall be applied in the dressing room in the presence of a Commission Representative and both contestants. Either contestant may waive his privilege of witnessing the bandaging of his opponents hands.

- No tape may be applied across the knuckles of any participant.

- The tape portion of the hand wrap must not extend past the top of the hand when a fist is made.

- Alternating (stacking) between tape and gauze is prohibited.

- The application of any liquid or substance to the hand wraps or bandages is prohibited.

- Report any violations immediately to the Dressing Room or Event Lead.

After observing the application of the wraps, the Inspector is to mark and sign the wraps with a felt-tip marker (on both sides of the hand) in such a way that if the wraps were later altered it would be recognizable. Once a participant's hands are wrapped, he or she must not leave the dressing room unless an Inspector escorts them.

Immediately after the contest ends, the Inspector is to observe the removal of the gloves in the ring, and carefully examine the wraps to ensure that they have not been altered. If the Inspector believes the wraps have been altered, he must immediately advise the Event Lead and not release the participant from his immediate supervision until the issue has been resolved.

## "Boxing Referee Rules and Guidelines for Championship Bouts" 2009

### Section 11. Bandages/Wrappings

The use of water or any liquid or material on any part of the handwrap is strictly prohibited.

Bandages will be adjusted in the dressing room in the presence of both contestants and a CSAC representative. All bandages/wrappings are to be signed off by a CSAC representative. Either contestant may waive his privilege of witnessing the bandaging/wrapping of his opponent's hands.

## Section 12. Regulatory Bandages/Wrappings

Bandages will not exceed the following restrictions:

One winding of **surgeon's adhesive tape**, not over one and one-half inches wide, placed directly on the hand to protect that part of the hand near the wrist. Said tape may cross the back of the hand twice but not extend within one-inch of the knuckles when the fist is clenched to make a fist. See figure CI-68

Contestants will use **soft surgical bandage** not over two inches wide, held in place by no more than ten yards of **surgeon's adhesive tape** for each hand. No more than thirty yards of **bandage** may be used to complete the wrappings for each hand. See figures CI-69 thru CI-72

When using championship rules, the use of up to 30 yards of gauze and 10 yards of tape is allowed on each hand upon approval by the Executive Officer. The gauze and tape must be applied in the same manner as previously noted.

- **Professional MMA Striker References and Rules**

### Professional MMA Striker

Licensed Professional MMA Strikers have the option of utilizing the gauze or tape. Since the gloves used in MMA events are so small, those that do use the gauze and/or tape only use it sparingly. Again, one can only use **Soft Surgical Bandage (Gauze)** and **Surgeon's Adhesive Tape (Tape).**

**All Professional MMA Strikers will adhere to the State Athletic Commissions Policy's listed from the Commissions:**

**"Professional Mixed Martial Arts Rules and Referee Guidelines" 2009**

### Section 9. Bandages

Bandages are optional.

Tape over the knuckles is prohibited.

If bandages are used, don't start handwrapping without an Inspector present.

Bandages will not exceed the following restrictions:

The use of water or any liquid or material on any part of the handwrap is strictly prohibited.

Bandages will be adjusted in the dressing room in the presence of both contestants and a Commission representative. All bandages/wrappings are to be signed off by a Commission representative. Either contestant may waive his privilege of witnessing the bandaging/wrapping of his opponent's hands.

One winding of **surgeon's adhesive tape**, not over one and one-half inches wide, placed directly on the hand to protect that part of the hand near the wrist. Said tape may cross the back of the hand twice but will not extend within one-inch of the knuckles when the hand is clinched to make a fist. See figure CI-73

Contestants will use **soft surgical bandage** not over two inches wide, held in place by no more than ten yards of **surgeon's adhesive tape** for each hand. No more than twenty yards of **bandage** may be used to complete the wrappings for each hand. See figures CI-74 thru CI-77

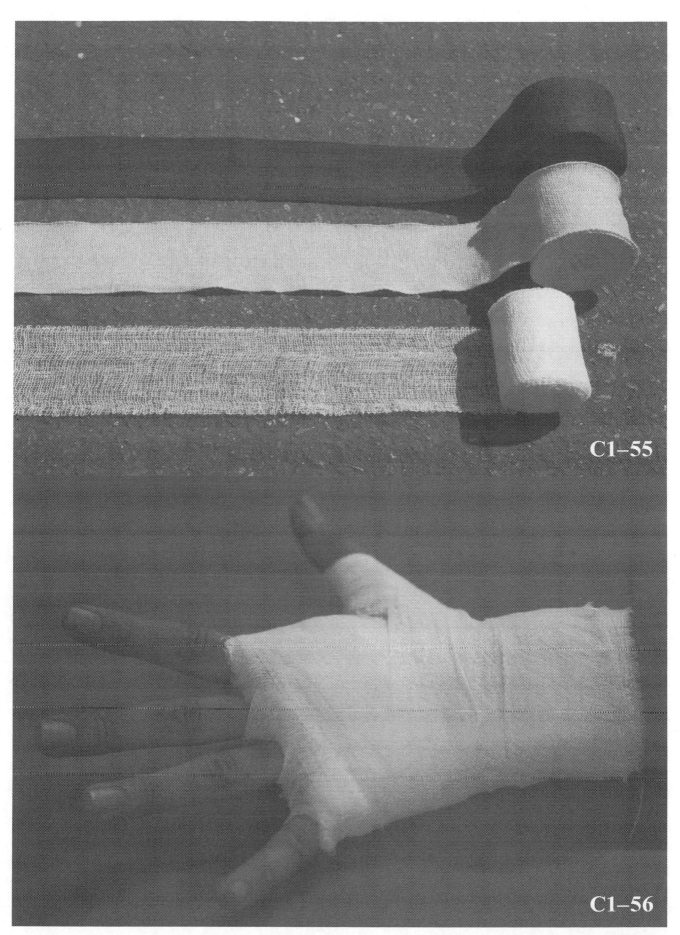

C1–55

C1–56

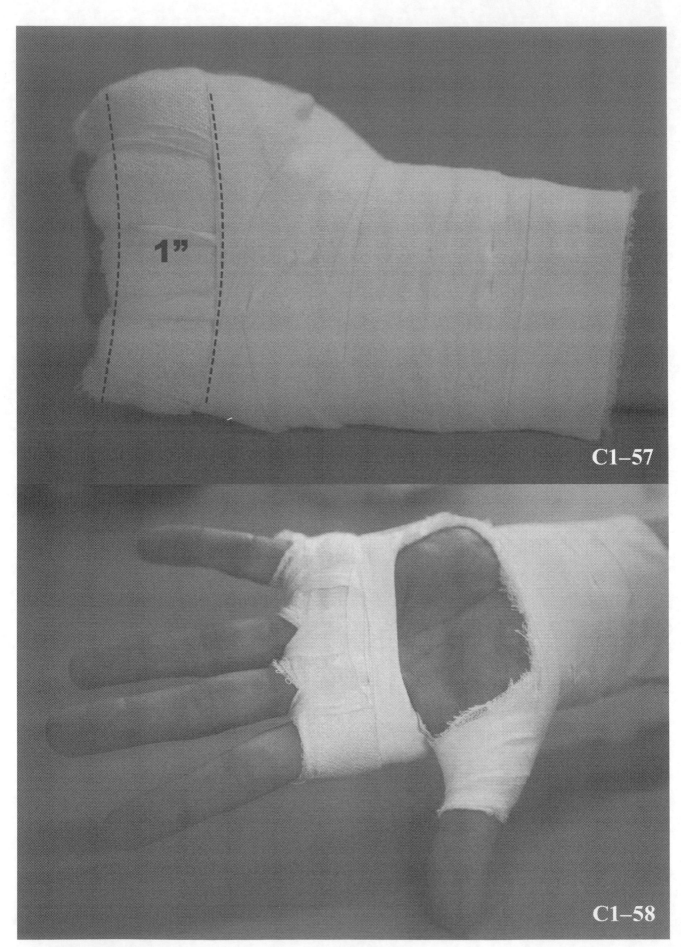

1"

C1–57

C1–58

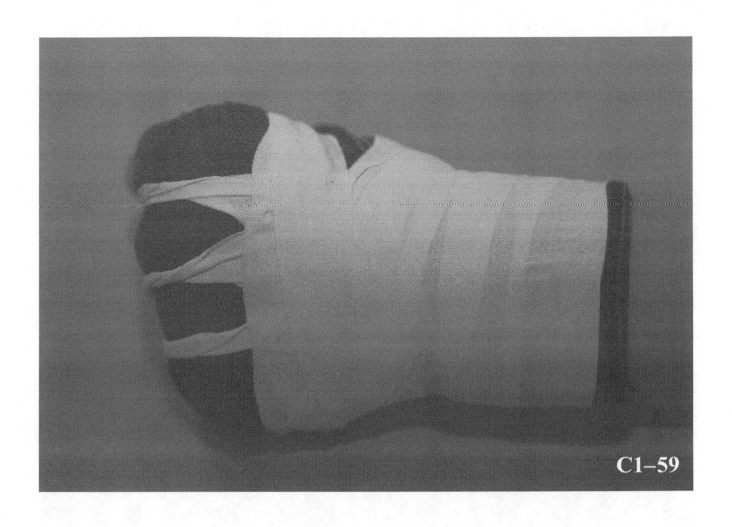

C1-59

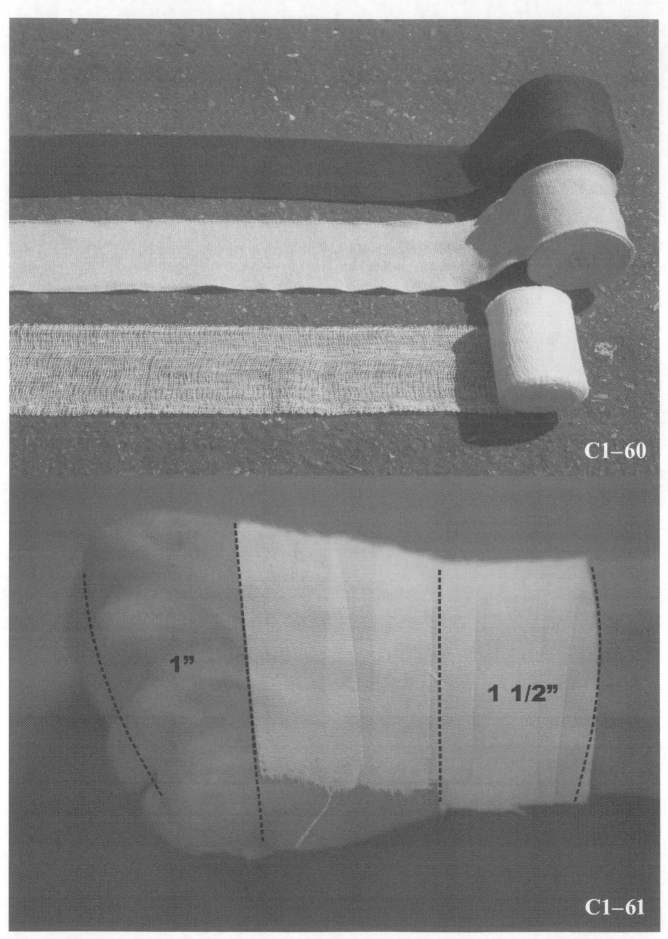

C1–60

1"

1 1/2"

C1–61

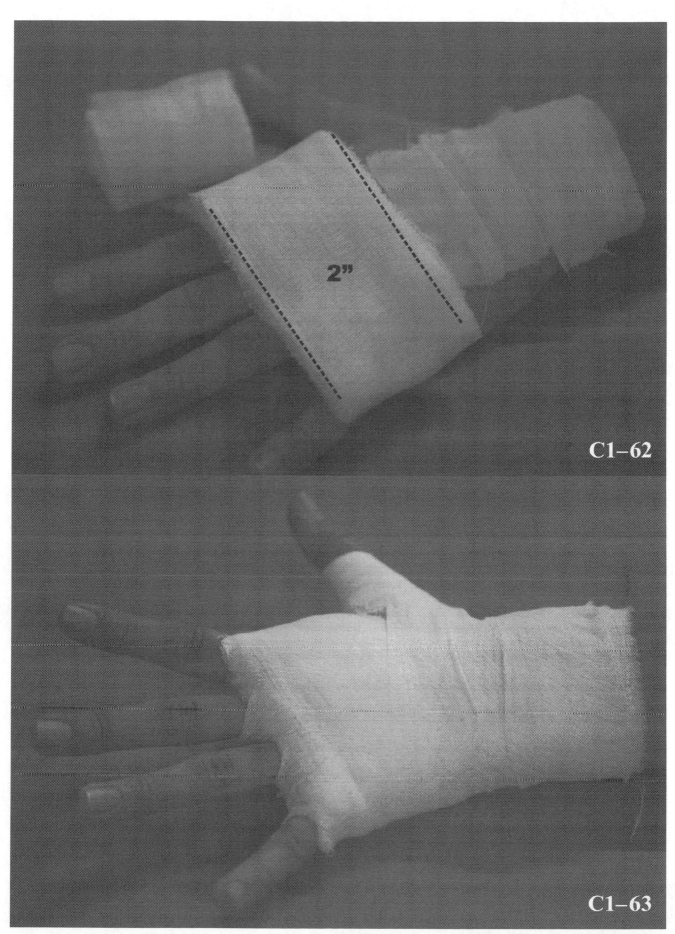

2"

C1–62

C1–63

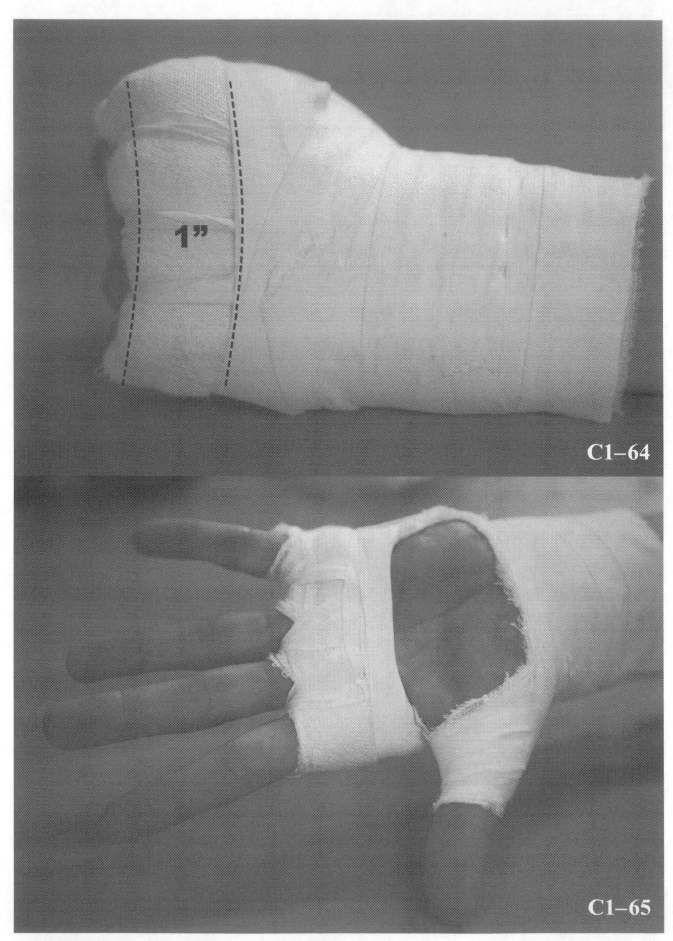

1"

C1–64

C1–65

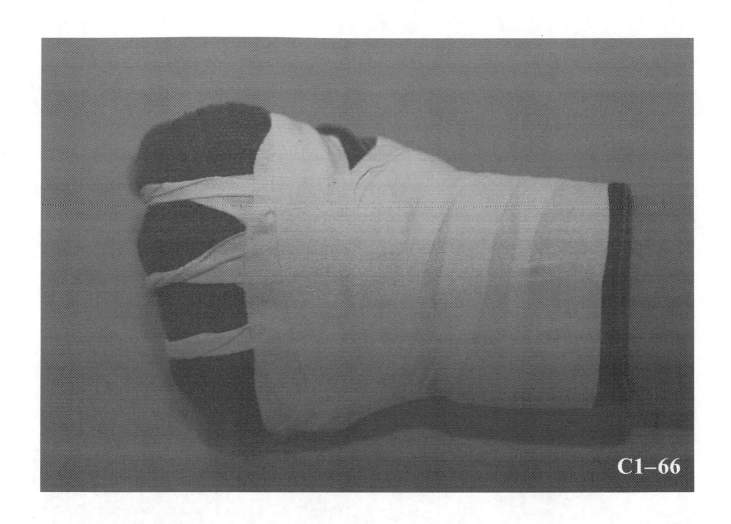

C1–66

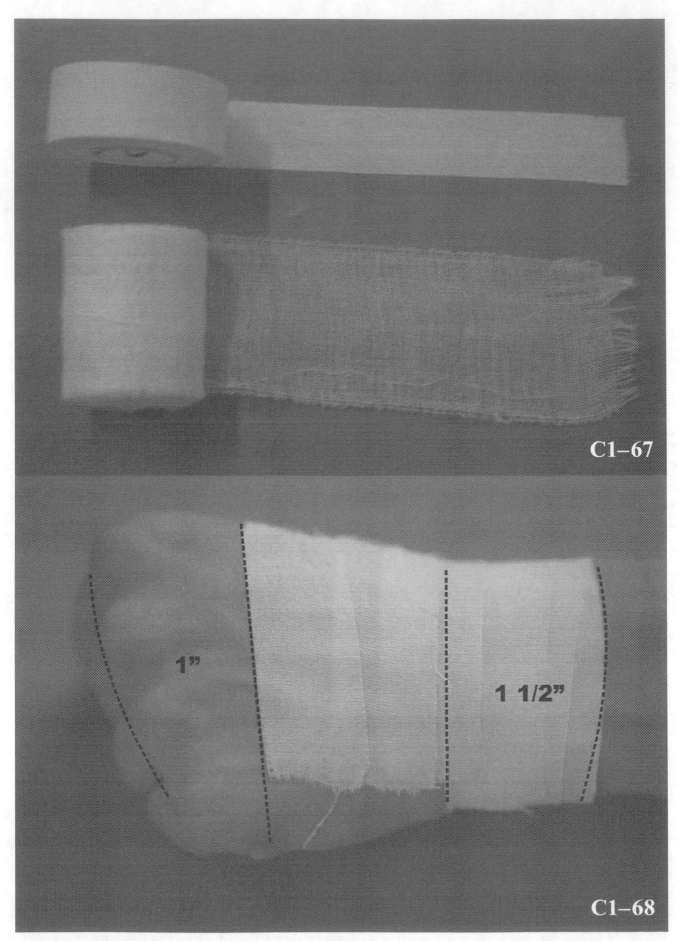

C1–67

1"

1 1/2"

C1–68

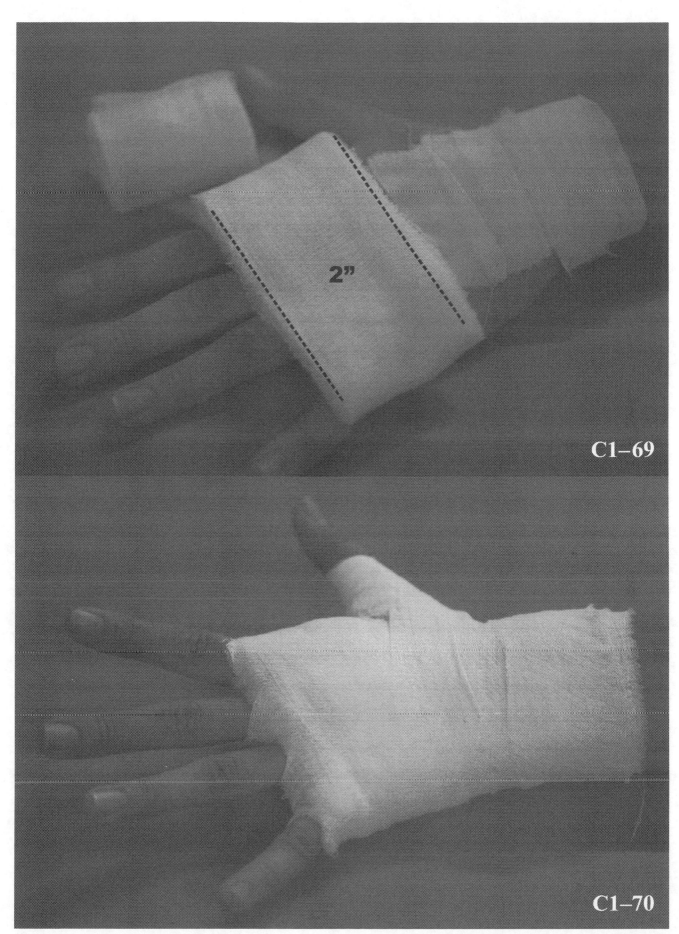

2"

C1–69

C1–70

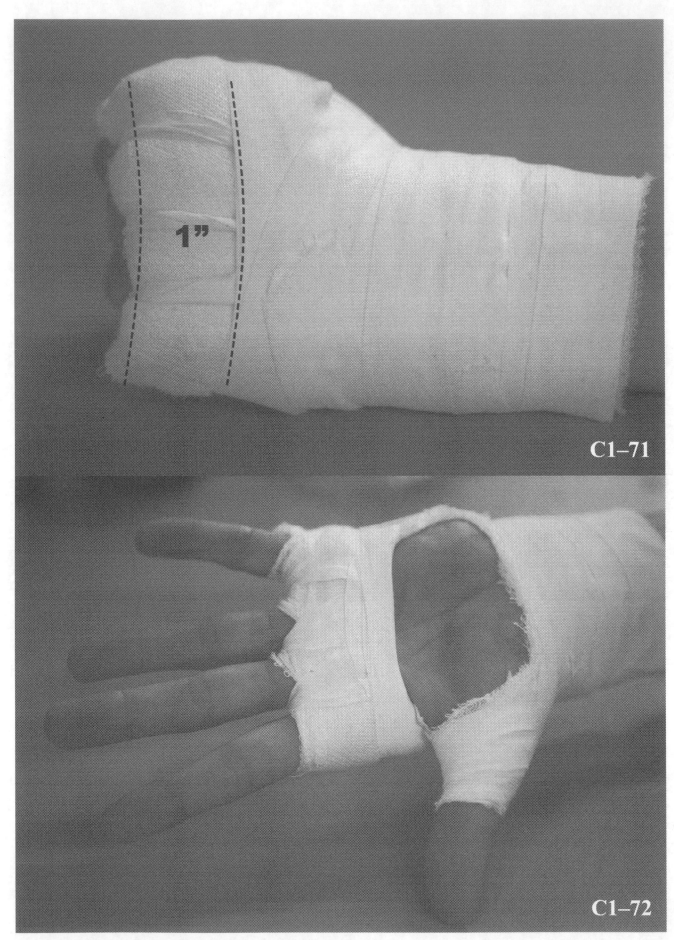

1"

C1–71

C1–72

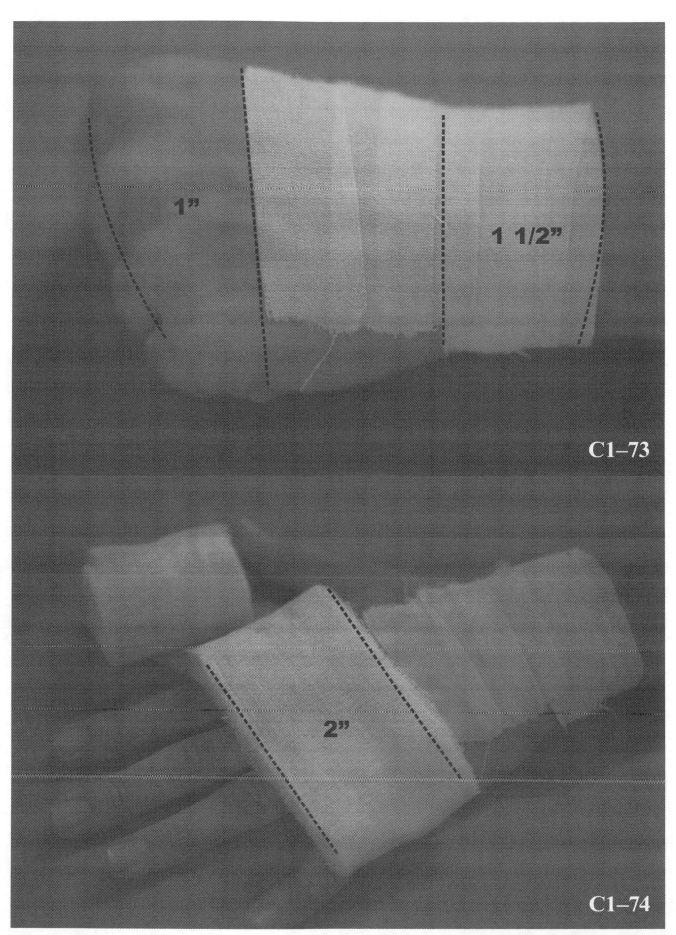

1"

1 1/2"

C1–73

2"

C1–74

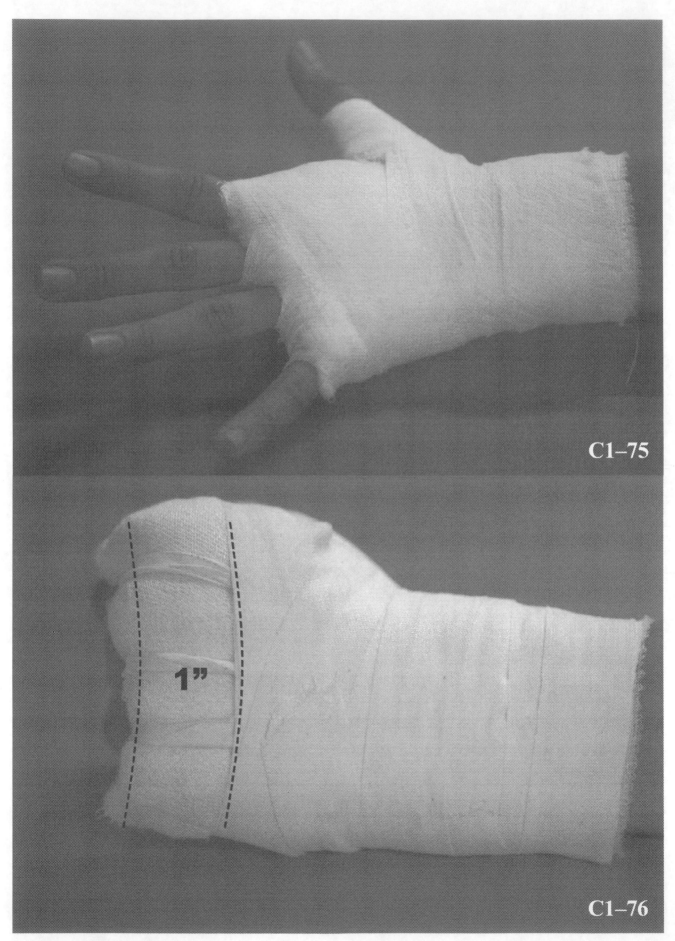

C1–75

1"

C1–76

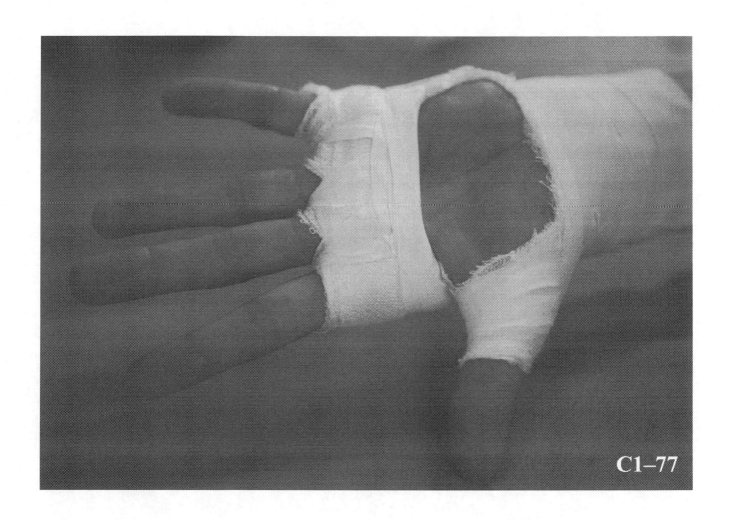

C1–77

# **<u>NOTES</u>**

# II POSITIONING

## Introduction

Let me explain the positioning concept. Boxing/striking is all about where you are positioned in order to strike and where to strike. No matter how tall or short an opponent is, you have only an arms length to reach them when striking with your hands or elbows. You want to practice getting the position for **long range** striking, **mid-range** striking, and up-**close** and personal striking. Most strikers, including Professional Boxers, want to be up-close and personal (**medium-close position**). Why stay that close if you can beat somebody down utilizing your **long-medium positions**, striking with power and control, making the fight easier for you? We will do all the above and have fun doing it too!

## Guard

For the **long-medium** range position, your hands should be held up just below your eyes and even with your cheeks, the arms starting from an L-shape. Your elbows and forearms should be in front of your midsection and held inside your body. Your legs should be shoulder width apart and the left foot/heel positioned in front of the back foot/toe. See figure CII-1

There are a few excellent reasons for having your guard in this position such as blocking punches, blocks and counters, parrying punches, faster hand speed. We'll get into that later in this book. If your opponent tries to get underneath you with their head, you can use your forearms to prevent his head from coming up and head butting you. Lean onto his body and move him one way or the other. This sets you up to throw a few strategically placed elbows.

This also helps maintain your mid-close position in order to hand them a better beating. If they grab you by the neck and try to land knees to your head or body, drive those elbows of yours into their knees and make them pay! You will be in a nice position to land uppercuts with your fist plus upper and cross elbows.

- **Long Range:** Extend your arm out as far as you can without locking the elbow. This range is for jabs, power punches, and combinations.
  See figure CII-2

- **Medium Range:** Your arms will be held in a wide V-shape. This position is for certain hooks, uppercuts, and the #4 jab (to be explained later).
  See figures CII-3 & CII-4

- **Close Range:** Your arms will be held in the L-shape. This is for short uppercuts, hooks, and elbows.
  See figures CII-5 & CII-6

- The **Shield** is an "Iron Mike" Tyson type of position it is used for in-fighting and is a very tight position of the arms and hands for the more explosive shots to the head and body. Place your elbows close to your body with your fists placed just below your eyes/cheeks. When you and your opponent are engaged in a war and are both firing away, keep your composure and an eye open in order to recognize spots to hit and positions to get into for an easy yet rousing display of infighting. You will be constantly moving and hitting your foe until he is unconscious or the referee stops the bout, whichever comes first. See figure CII-7

- **Safety Block** is what "Smokin Joe" Frazer and Ken Norton had perfected. The safety block was one of the best guards back in the day. It is not used as frequently as before and therefore is unfamiliar to many followers of fistiana. It consists of bringing both hands and arms into use. Fold the right forearm across the face with the nose and chin fitting snugly into the crook of the elbow. The left arm is held directly across the front of the body, the upper arm covering the heart and left ribs. The forearm and hand with the palm opened and turned in protects the pit of the stomach and right ribs. This block can be made more as a "safety" by bending the stomach inward as you carry the arms into position. See figure CII-8

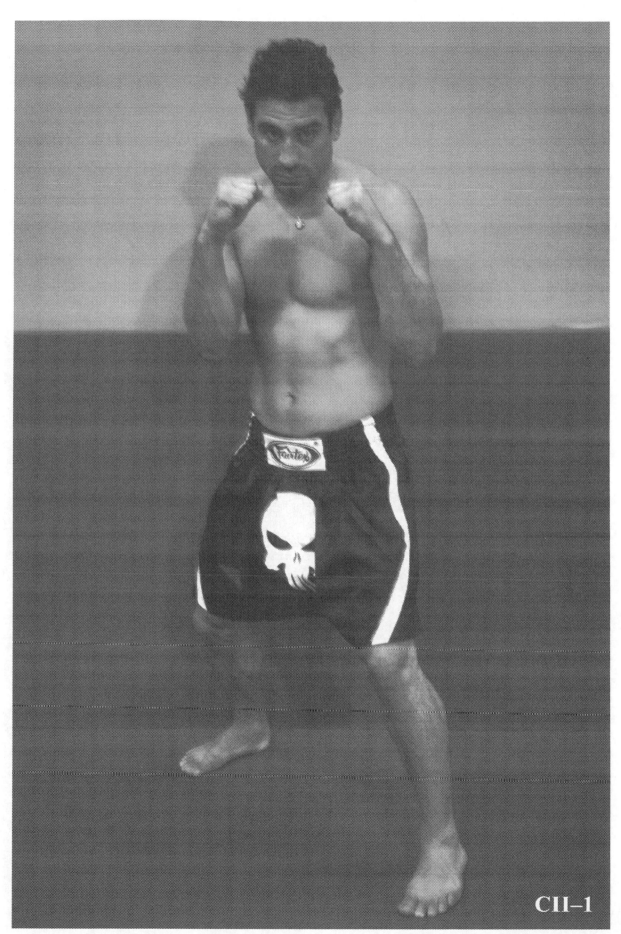

**CII-1**

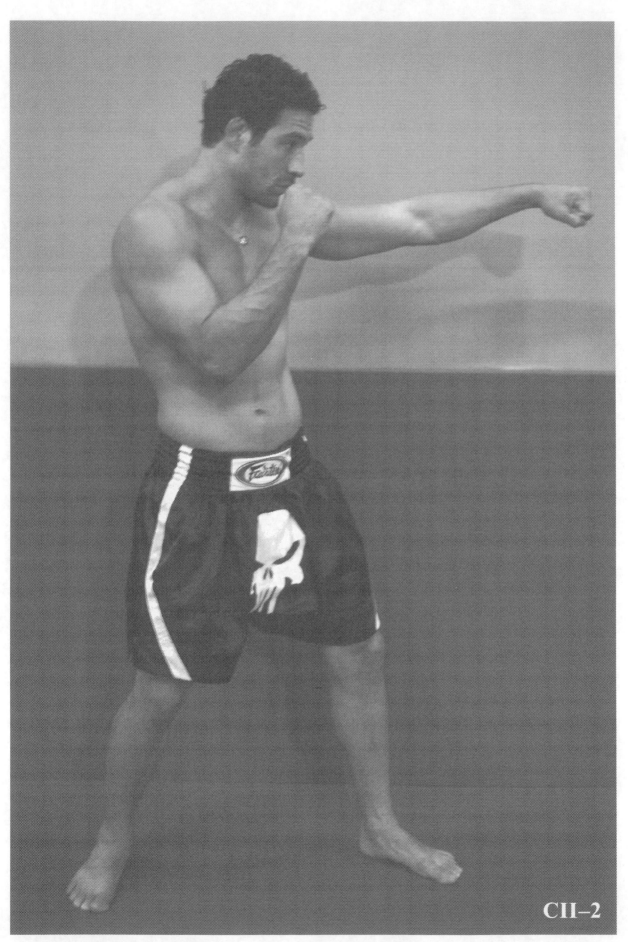

CII–2

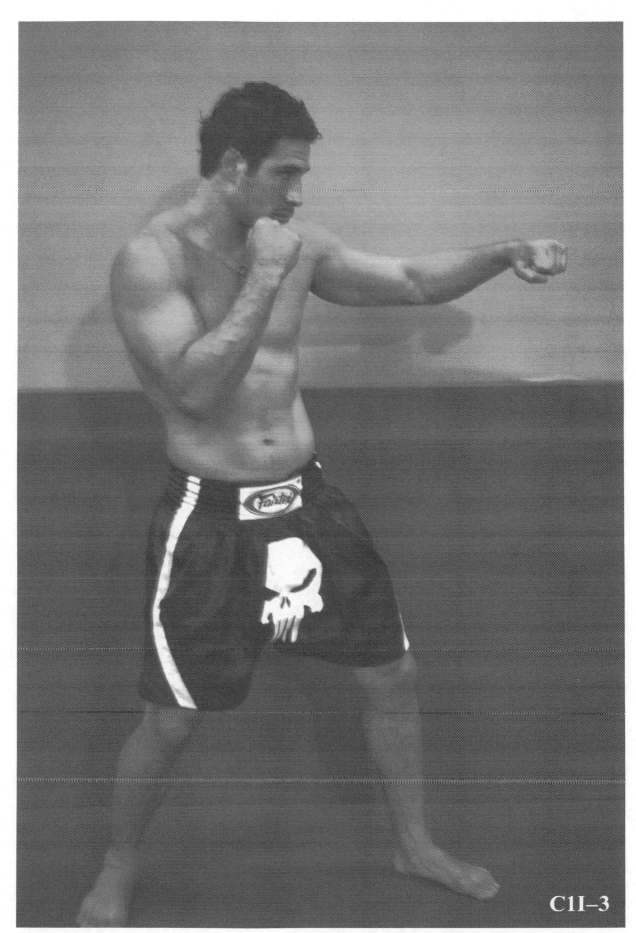

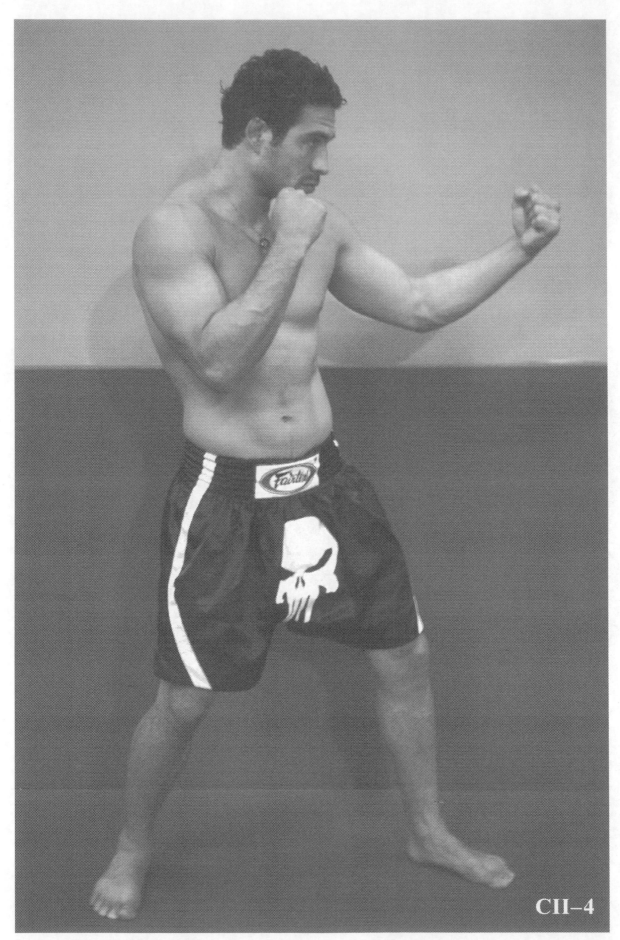

CII–4

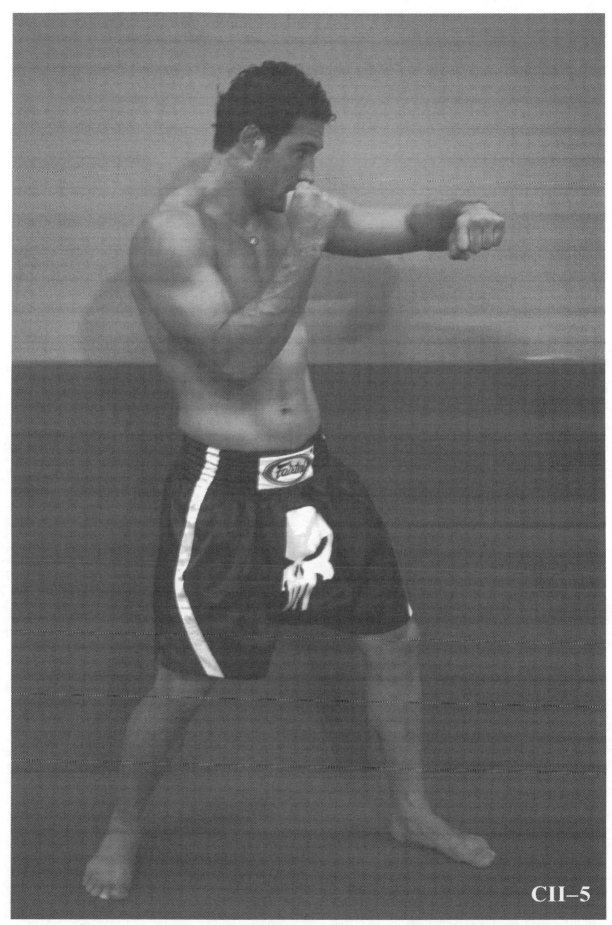

CII–5

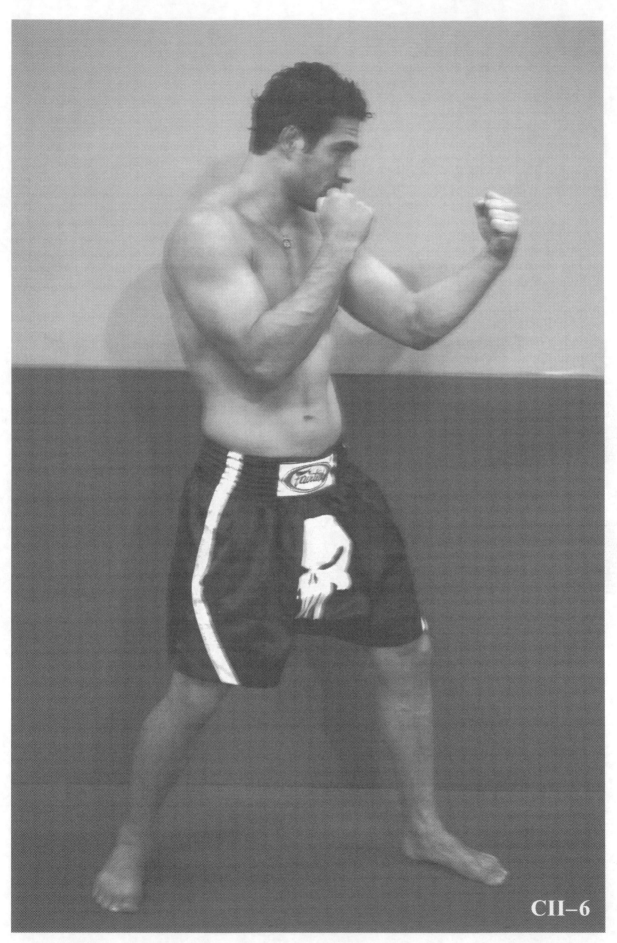

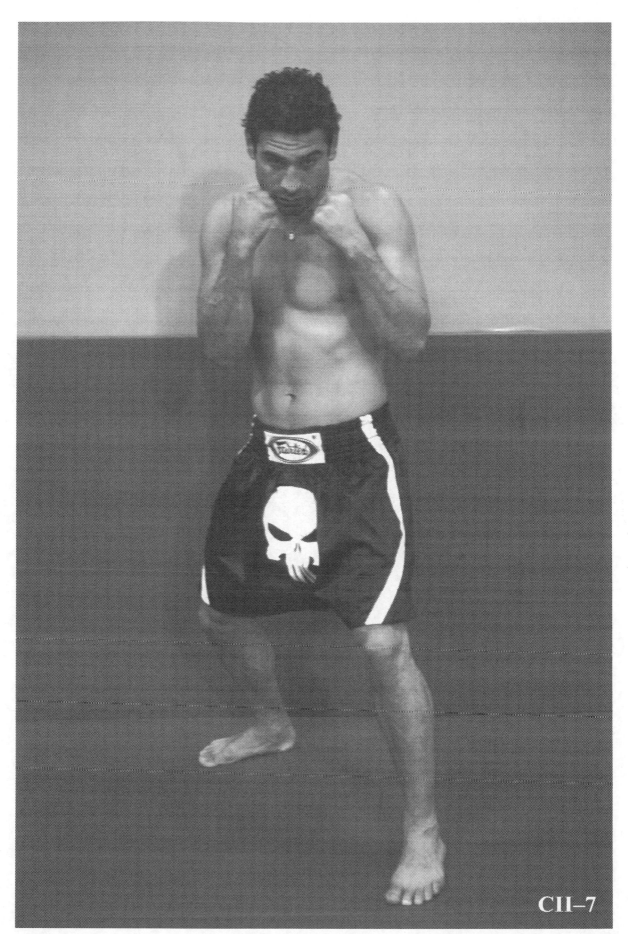

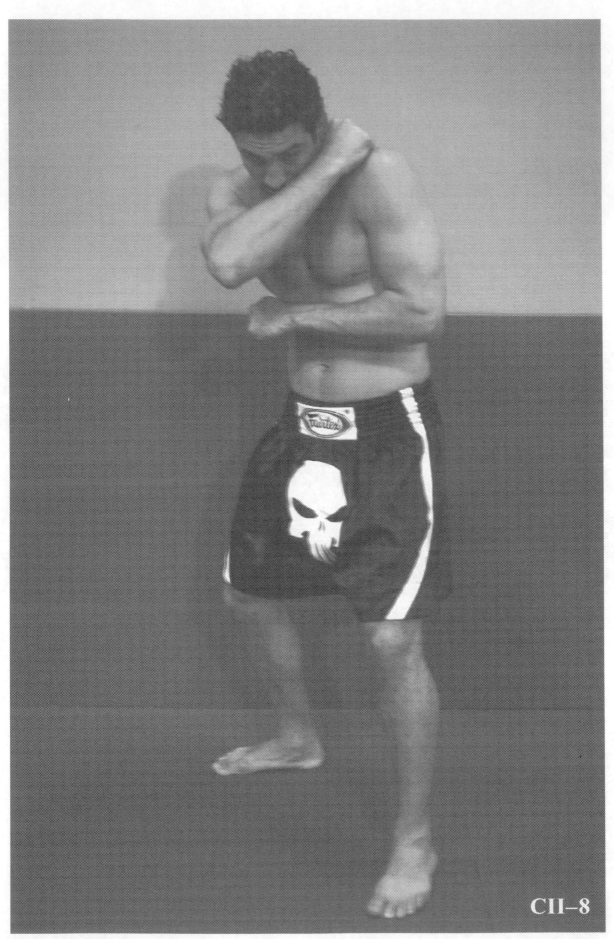

## III DEFENSES

### Introduction

I cannot say enough about defense. There have been great defensive fighters such as Muhammad Ali, Wilfredo Benitez, Joe Frazer, Roberto Duran, and Mike Tyson to name a few. Each had their own unique method of defense. Guarding the body is a valuable piece of knowledge which is seldom done justice by writers on the "Manly Art."

All fighters should take great pride and care to learn how to protect themselves quickly and effectively from an attack. Hitting without being hit is an art unto itself. Growing up watching the great champions mentioned above was such a thrill. Their movement and grace was what made them not just champions but great champions. I will try and do as much justice to the art of defense as possible in the next few pages.

One rule of thumb on the defensive positioning is, moving your chin over your knee or staying in between your knees as in the soft blocking. Remember, your chin should never go past your knees. If you do this, you will stretch your opposite leg out and be out of position for a quick and safe recovery or counter.

### Four phases to the Defensive moves

- The actual **Defensive** move; make them miss

- The **Position** for the counter-punch; make them miss and be in position to make them pay by countering

- The **Counter-Punch;** make them miss and make them pay

- Then **Countering the Counter;** being able to hit without being hit.

Never stay in one place once you've thrown your combinations. After striking, move to another position offensively or defensively.

For example:

1.) Take one step backwards and be ready to move back in.

2.) Side step to either side usually a 2-step.

3.) Stay in position and utilize your defenses to get into another offensive position.

4.) Jab out, not getting too far from your victim, and leaving you in a better position for kicks, punches, knees, and/or elbows.

**Four Defensives:**

- **Slipping** side to side towards hips.

  Slipping **side to side** refers to slipping to the outside or inside of the punch, moving to the sides towards the hips, **not leaning**. This defense works best when the opponents reach is the same length as yours or they have a tendency to lean or step in with their punches. See figure CIII-1

- **Slipping** in, leaning in towards your knees.

  Slipping towards your opponent's body or your knees refers to moving (**leaning**) your head forward of the punch thrown. If your opponent is taller or has a longer reach than yours, this is what you will have to do in order to compensate for your shorter reach. See figure CIII-2

- **Bobbing and Weaving;** both side to side and leaning forward.

  **Bob** or duck away from the punch and towards your left or right knee for some hard positions. **Weave** or duck back out to another position over your other knee. These defenses work similarly to the side to side slipping and the leaning forward mentioned above. See figures CIII-3 thru CIII-5

- **Blocks and Parries**

  **Soft-blocking** means keeping your hands up and catching or blocking punches while having your chin centered between your knees. Counter with fast punches as soon as you block the punch coming at you. This will help get your timing down and frustrate your opponent because every time they throw a punch at you, you're hitting them. Blocking is unmistakably the first in importance and the most frequently adopted means of meeting a lead punch. Blocking, in most cases, should be done with as little effort as possible but when an opponent puts considerable force into their blow, it is advisable to meet it with sufficient power to prevent your guard from being driven back into your face or body. See figures CIII-6 & CIII-7

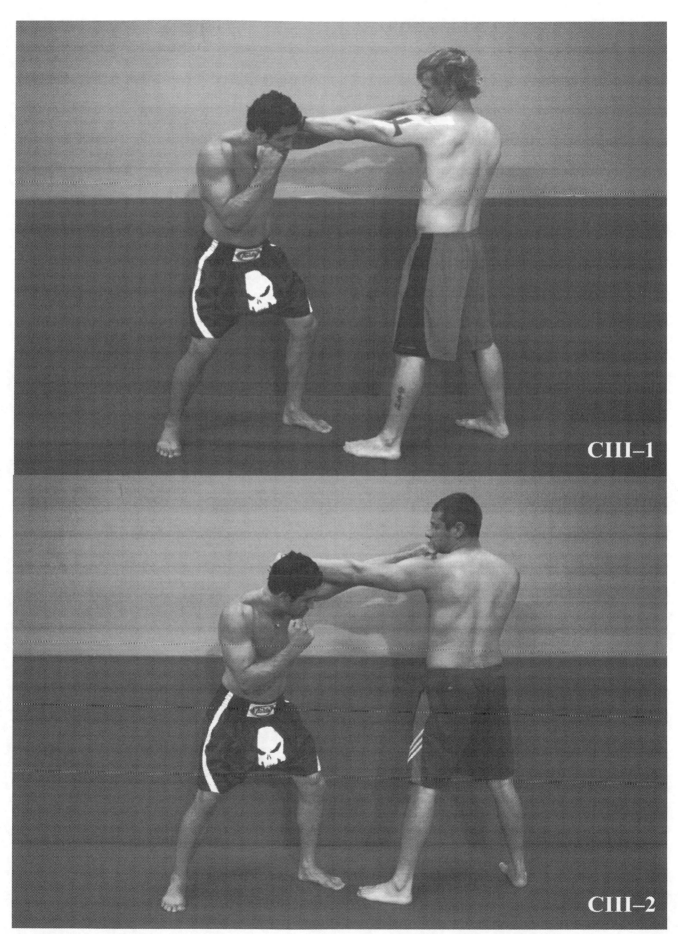

CIII–1

CIII–2

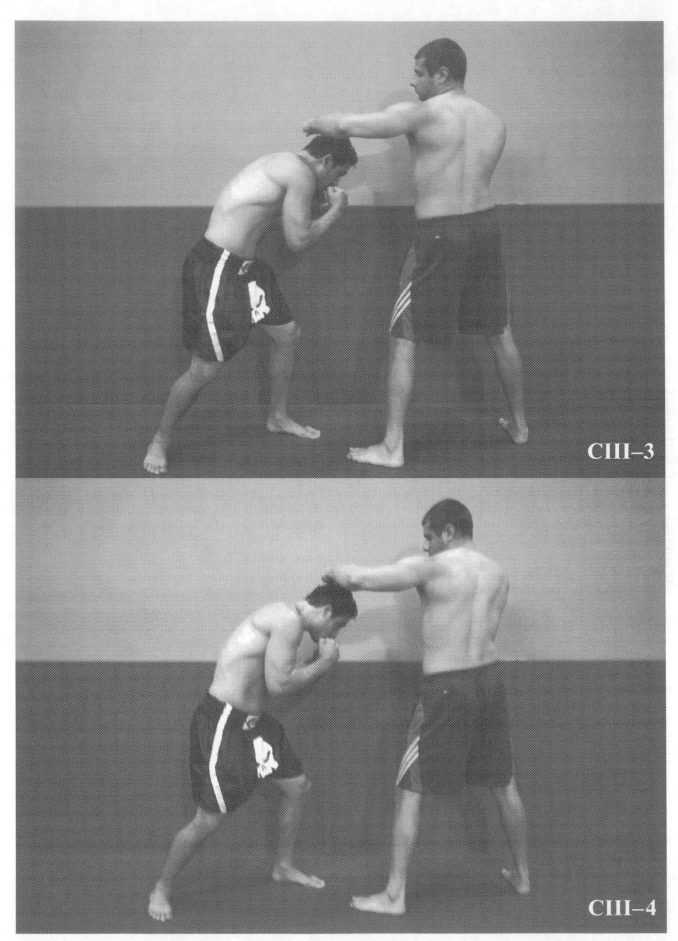

CIII–3

CIII–4

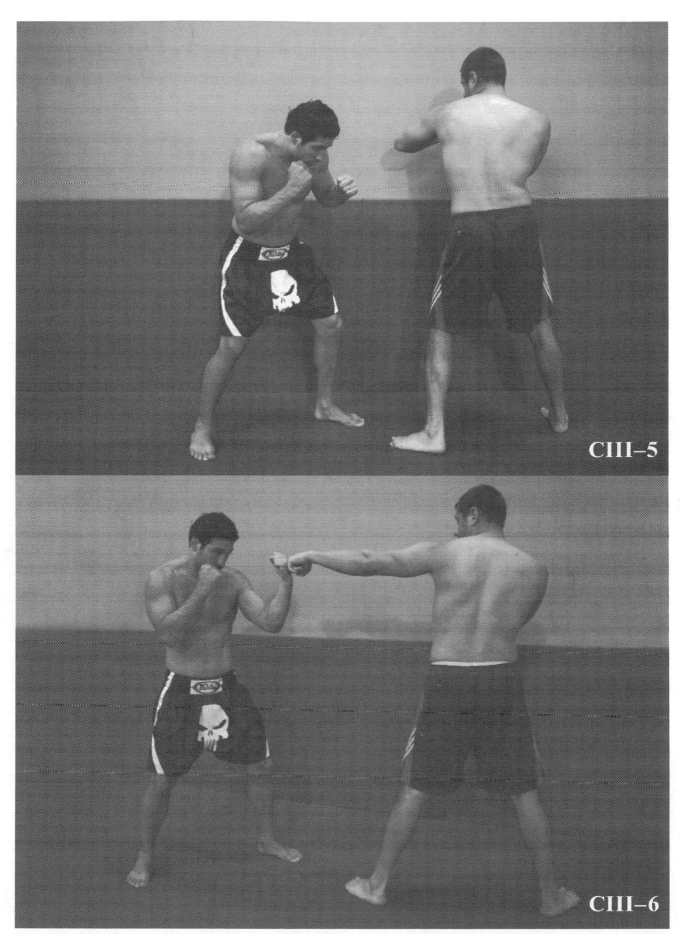

CIII–5

CIII–6

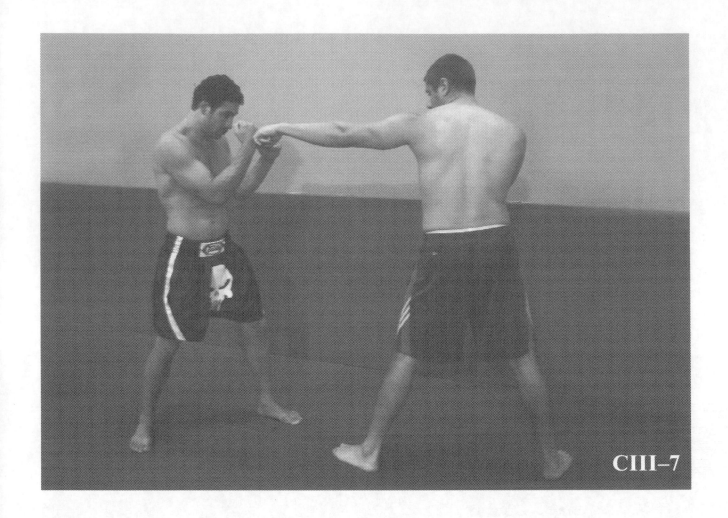

CIII–7

**Hard-blocking** is the art of getting into a *hard* punching position. First of all, you must be strong enough to get into this position and hold it in order to get the maximum power out of it. The hard-block requires putting up your shield arm (fist positioned in front of or just below your nose) and leaning into the punch being thrown. Position yourself into the hard punching position, having your chin over either of your knees (depending on which arm is the lead), body low and set, keeping your eyes on your opponent, then fire away! With your forearm in front of your face, the opponent will try and go around your arm and when he does or if he tries, strike with a hard, powerful straight punch. This punch can be to the head or body and from long-medium range or even a full step away, just stepping in with the punch.
See figure CIII-8

Always aim for something you know you'll hit, such as the body, wrist, or below the chin!

**Safety Block** is what "Smokin Joe" Frazer and Ken Norton had perfected. The safety block was one of the best guards back in the day. It is not used as frequently as before and therefore is unfamiliar to many followers of fistiana. It consists of bringing both hands and arms into use. Fold the right forearm across the face with the nose and chin fitting snugly into the crook of the elbow. The left arm is held directly across the front of the body, the upper arm covering the heart and left ribs. The forearm and hand with the palm opened and turned in protects the pit of the stomach and right ribs. This block can be made more as a "safety" by bending the stomach inward as you carry the arms into position.
See figure CIII-9

**Parry** is another method of defense which proves troublesome to an opponent. Parrying consists of stopping your opponent's punches before they are shot. By having your hands in the guard position, just place your open or closed glove over your opponent's glove before they throw a punch at you. Notice any slight movement of the hands, shoulders, or head before a punch is thrown. Once you notice movement coming from either hand, parry the shot before it is thrown. This will not only tire an opponent's arms and hands, it will also discourage them. To add more salt to the wound, parry and counter punch with a nice solid shot to the head or body.
See figures CIII-10 & CIII-11

# NOTES

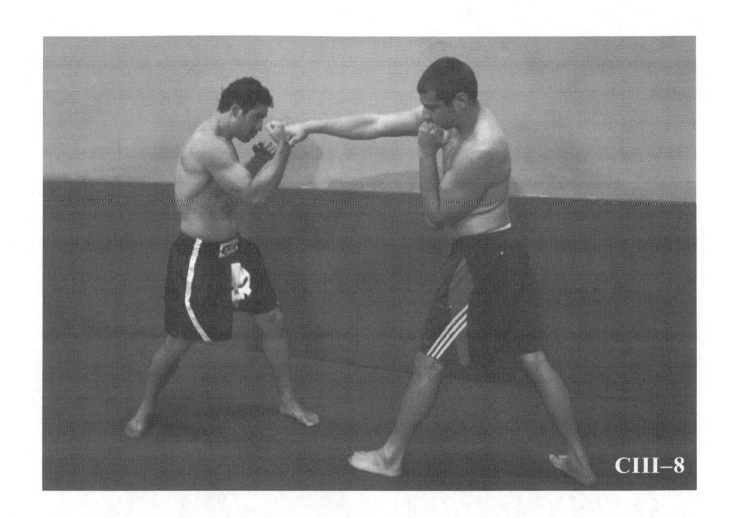

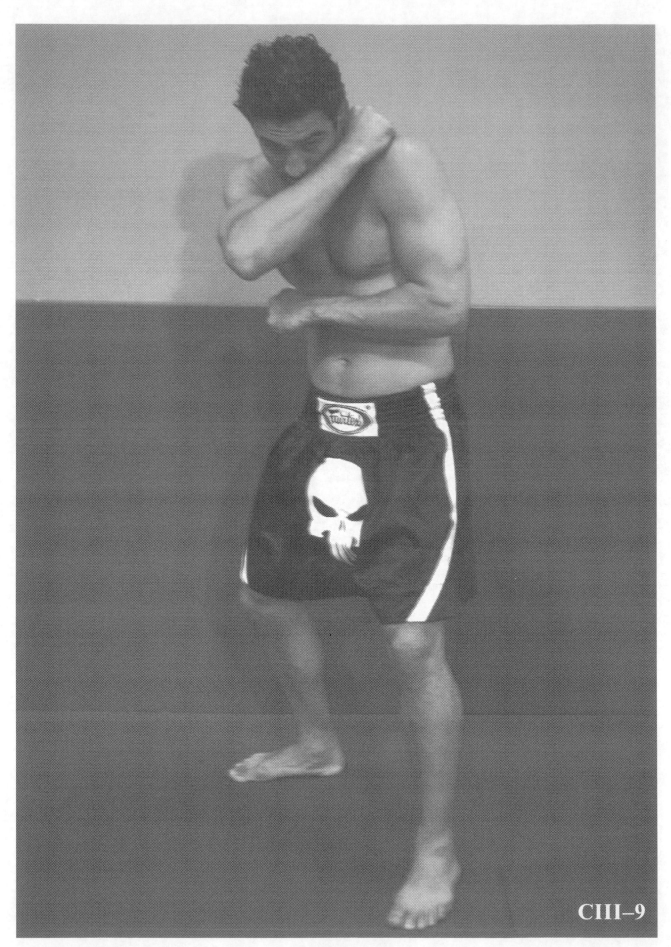

CIII–9

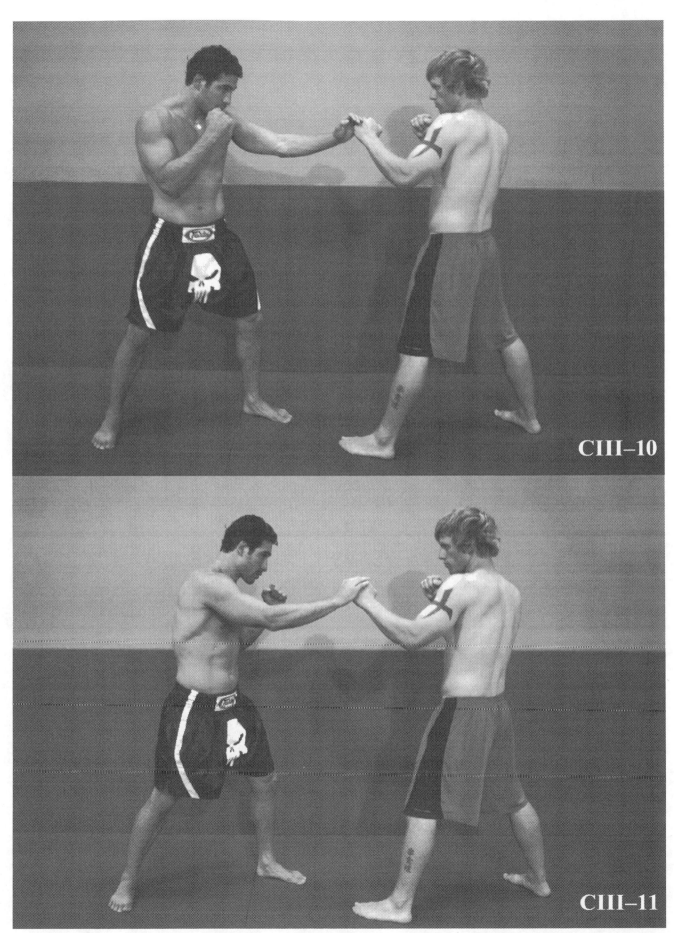

CIII–10

CIII–11

## Footwork

**The Value of Footwork:** One of the prime essentials to success in the ring or cage is the clever and strategic use of the feet. Many fights are lost due to weariness or some other cause where a fighter makes a false move. A fight may be lost because the fighter is unable to avoid punishment or because bad maneuvering prevents him from getting into position to hit his opponent at opportune moments.

## Footwork

First of all, use the balls of your feet and ankles to move. Some times when moving you will step with your lead foot and slide your back foot (step and slide). Be sure to keep the distance between your legs the same, always leaving yourself ready to punch or take a punch.

The size of your foot dictates your footwork! One step is the size of your foot, whether it's moving in, out, or side to side. Never step more than your full foot size.
See figures CIII-12 & CIII-13

You can use smaller steps when stalking or moving from the long-medium range to the medium-short range by just taking a ½ step.

Side-stepping is an important means of defense as well, especially when used in conjunction with the slipping, bobbing, weaving, or blocking. Add a counter or two and you have the making of a nice piece of art. The motion and fluidity of the movement are very impressive to your fans and the judges. More importantly, good fluid footwork will confuse the hell out of your opponent!

You also have pivots that are very nice when used correctly. Push off the mobile foot and pivot on the stationary foot, keeping the distance the same every time you settle. This sets you up to be in a better position to punch.

Faster and evasive (or as I like to call it, <u>persuasive</u>) footwork is effective for getting your opponent out of their zone and into following you like a sheep to slaughter. This footwork requires moving side to side and in and out, getting your opponent to follow you. You can utilize the jabs, fakes, and feints to achieve better positioning for beating your victim down. You must keep your body centered on your opponent, staying in your zone. Kicks, knees, elbows, and punches will follow.
See figures CIII-14 & CIII-15

If you are getting tired or you need to re-evaluate your opponent do not stand in front of them. Instead, you can use back peddling or shuffling out of the range of your opponent's punches or strikes.

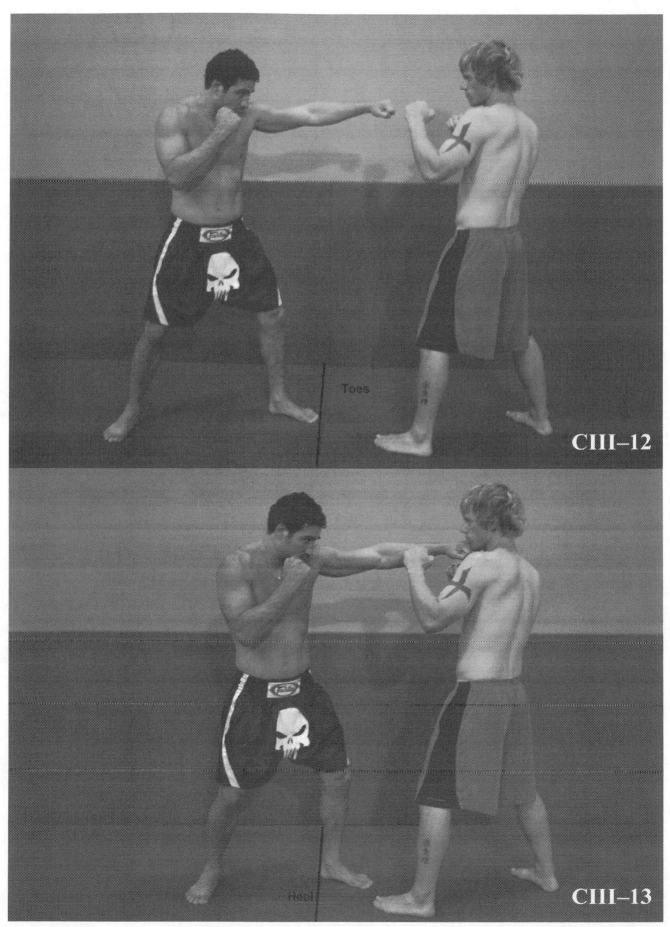

CIII–12

CIII–13

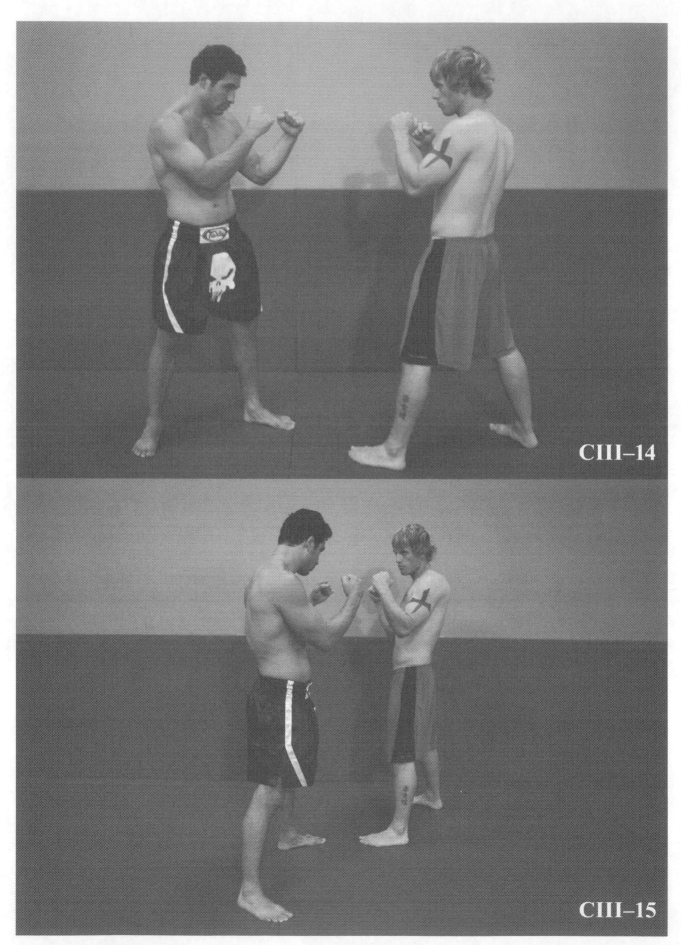

CIII–14

CIII–15

**Defensive Combinations, Counters, & Drills**

- **Defensive Combinations and Counters**

Mix up the defenses at all times so that you are not setting up a pattern. This keeps your opponent always trying to guess your next move while you are setting them up for your **counter punches**, **combinations**, or **power punches**. **Examples** of the defensive combos are: slip outside a jab, then block a right hand with your right hand, then deliver a solid #7 jab to his chin (it will be detailed in the Jabs Chapter). Bob in, weave out, and then bob back, setting up for a nice left hook to the head or body. With your footwork, step and slip to your opponent's right side, bob out, and deliver a straight right to his or her chin. The main idea is to set your opponent up to hit him without getting hit back.

- **Defensive drills: Puncher-Punchy/Combinations/Countering/Stalking (Bull-dog Defense):**

The defensive work we do is for both the **Puncher (offense)** and the **Punchy (defense).**

When practicing with a partner, the **Puncher** will work their offensive positioning by utilizing their 7 jabs (explained later), combinations, and positions. Punch with power and control while controlling the pace. The **Puncher** will also be practicing their **defensive combinations**.

The **Punchy** will work their **defensive combinations** to get into some strong offensive **countering** positions, attempting to control the pace as well. To push the envelope they will add their **Bull-Dog defense** to the exercise in the form of **Stalking.**

The **Stalker (Bull-dog Defense)** will methodically pursue their opponent utilizing their offenses and defenses. The footwork will be either one full foot step, which is the maximum you will need, or the ½ step. The **Punchy** will move forward, side to side, forward and backward, bobbing and weaving, slipping, hard blocking, and soft blocking to control the pace. While stalking, they will also be **counter** punching up, down, in, and out, beating down their opponent.

In the beginning the **Puncher** will start slowly, not trying to hit their opponent hard, but rather focusing on and practicing their correct form and positions. The **Punchy** does not counter, but instead, practices their defenses and getting into their solid/hard punching positions working at around 50-75%. If both are comfortable with their skills there will be full contact punching and countering (with power and control!). Let the fun begin!

When by yourself, practice in front of a **mirror** by placing a piece of tape about the width of a fist by 12 inches long, with the bottom at chin level on the mirror. Your head and body should be placed directly in the middle of the tape. Practice the slip to the outside of the tape; you should be able to see your whole head (face) in the mirror.
See figure CIII-16

Now, move your head to the other side, continuing to practicing your slipping. Next, practice bobbing and weaving making sure you are dropping under the lower end of the tape. Again, you should be able to see your whole head when you come up.

Practice the blocking exercise and then the footwork.  Once proficient, start mixing them up by slipping and stepping, or bobbing and stepping etc...  You want to develop muscle memory for these movements.  When you feel comfortable with your movements, start **countering** at the head and body after every move.  Practice, practice, and more practice is what it will take to perfect the defense and countering you will need to become a champion.  See figure CIII-17

Start slow and easy, getting the correct positions down.  After a while get mean, move and hit fast and hard, utilizing power and control.  Know where you are hitting at all times! (This will be mentioned again in the mirror work section)

### How to protect your stomach without blocking (breathing)

The Solar Plexus (stomach) punch, when delivered correctly, has a telling effect on an opponent.  When delivered to the soft/weak parts of the stomach and at the precise time, it will disable your opponent and allow you to go home early.  It can tire and wear down an opponent, or hurt and stop them in their tracks.

To protect yourself from this damage you will need to practice short inhalations through the nose and exhaling in short puffs through the nose or mouth.  This causes your stomach muscles to rebound outward, continuously inflating and deflating, protecting your stomach from any unexpected blows that you may receive.

This form of breathing, if carried out throughout the rounds, has several advantages.  First, it keeps your head clear and prevents dizziness when you are rocked with head punches.  By controlling your breathing you are also prepared for any unexpected body blows.  It keeps your wind in and stores up energy that otherwise would be expelled in natural breathing.

 If you need to clear your breath and/or need more air, step or move away from your opponent, far enough so that you are not in harms way and take a deep breath.  Exhale in a slow smooth fashion, lowering your heart rate and thus clearing your head.  If practiced throughout the bout you will find that you are as fresh in the closing round as in the opening.  You will also need to do this in between rounds.  Of course this does not prevent punishment, but will lessen it a great deal.

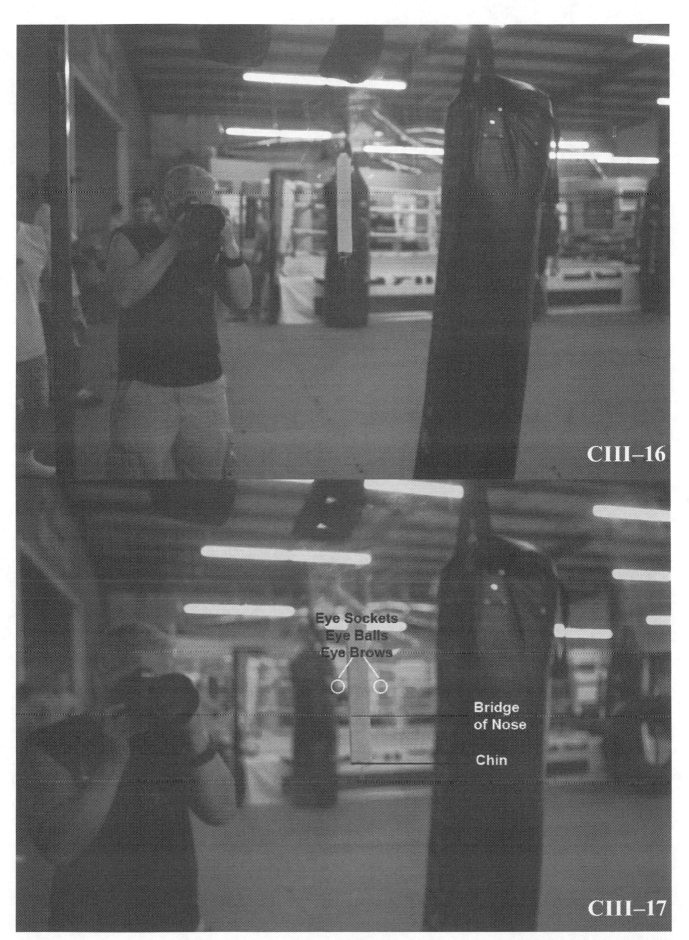

**CIII–16**

Eye Sockets
Eye Balls
Eye Brows

Bridge
of Nose

Chin

**CIII–17**

# NOTES

# IV STRIKE ZONES

## Introduction

When striking an opponent there are up, down, in, and out zones you want to hit.  You don't have to look at where you are going to strike, but you do need to know where it is you are striking.  A well placed shot will stop an opponent more than just hitting hard all the time. It will also take less time, energy, and effort.

- **Up**; is towards the head

- **Down**; is towards the body and legs

- **Up and in**; is inside the head area such as the eyeballs, eyebrow, nose, lips, and the sweet spot; the tip of the chin.

- **Up and out**; are the temple, the ear drum, below the ear lobe; behind the jaw joint, the jaw line, and the eyebrow.

- **Down and in**; is inside the elbow area along the lower rib cage, and the middle stomach, and front & inner thigh

- **Down and out**; is the lower-outer rib cage just above the hip bone and below the elbow, plus inside the elbow towards the stomach and again along the rib cage, and front & outer thigh

- As a MMA Striker, beat the **inside, outside and front of the thigh** for those taller opponents you need to break down.
  See figures CIV-1 & CIV-2

An added bonus for MMA fighters is that you can also strike the legs, arms (both inside and outside), and use elbows.  The elbows are the most under- utilized weapons an MMA fighter has.  The elbows are the hardest bone on the human body and can cause the most injury if used correctly.  Use the elbows to strike anywhere legal, though on the head is preferred since it will cause vicious cuts and bleeding.

**Practice knowing where you are striking at all times, striking the (weak) soft parts of the upper and lower body.**

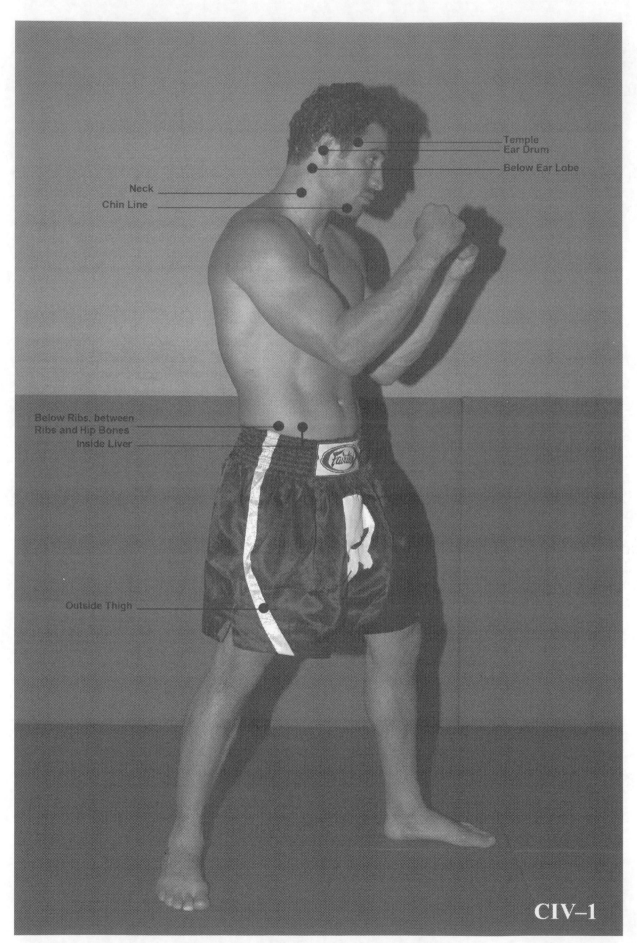

Temple
Ear Drum
Below Ear Lobe
Neck
Chin Line
Below Ribs, between
Ribs and Hip Bones
Inside Liver
Outside Thigh

CIV–1

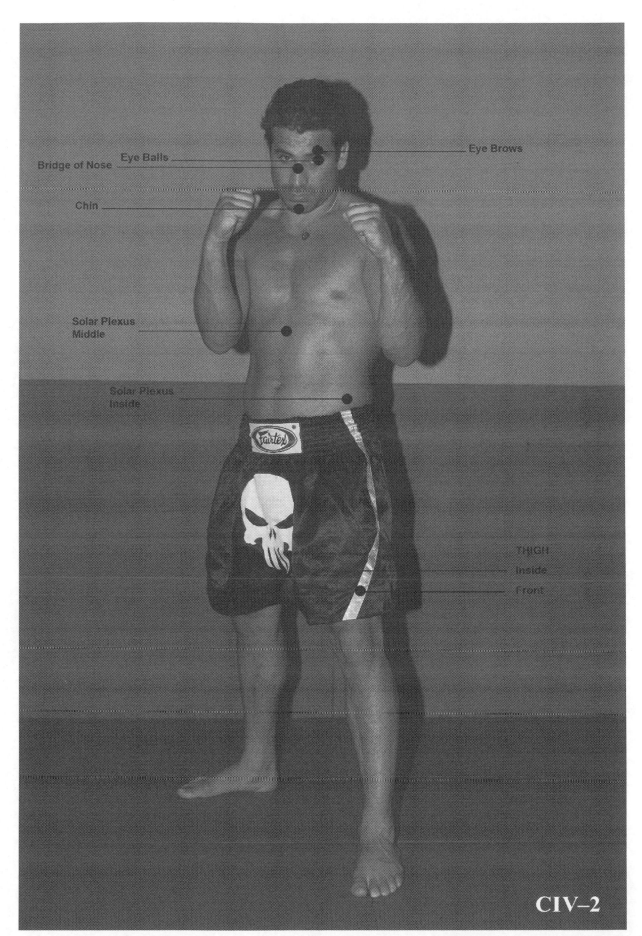

Bridge of Nose

Eye Balls

Eye Brows

Chin

Solar Plexus
Middle

Solar Plexus
Inside

THIGH

Inside

Front

**CIV–2**

# NOTES

# V OFFENSE

## Introduction

Most fighters have a specific punch that works for them. "Smokin Joe" Frazier had the left hook to the head or body. That was it; he had no right hand at all. Pepino Cuevas had a left hook as well although his was better for the body than the head. George Foreman had the upper hooks with either hand. Muhammad Ali had hand speed and combinations but did not have a straight knockout punch. He would beat them down with his speed and accuracy, eventually defeating them with more combinations. Mike Tyson would knock them out with either hand from all angles.

What I'm getting at is that all of these men were famous World Champion Boxers and all of these men had a punch or punches that worked for them. What are your punch and/or punches? Work hard at the exercises in the previous chapters and get a feel for the punch that works the best for you and perfect it.

Next, work on another backup punch or combination to work into the favorite punch. Will it be a left or a right hand? Or will it be a hook, uppercut, or a straight punch? Will it be my favorite, a body shot? The goal is to find what works for you and then find more weapons to add to your arsenal. Again, remember that there are the two ways to get into the perfect punching position; utilizing your defenses and/or offenses.

## Jabs

## Introduction

Jabs, if used correctly, can make a fight so much easier for you and will allow you to dictate the pace. Use your jabs in combinations; punching with authority, accuracy, power, and control. Always change speed, power, direction, and position. Deliver your jab to the nose, eye socket, body, lip, eye brow, arms, and hands. You want to have your opponents mind on the jab in order to keep them off balance and set them up for the power punches, including nice combinations of kicks, knees, elbows, and take downs.

### The 7-Jabs of Champions

1. The **Larry Holmes Jab** is for a taller striker. You will be in a ready position, hands up, right or left power hand set, no stepping in or out, just being at the ready. Throw the jab and be set to land a heavy power punch or a fast punch followed by a power punch. The jab will need to be direct with power and control.
   See figure CV-1

2. The **Mike Tyson Jab** is for a shorter striker. You will step in when jabbing and/or slipping; step and jab, or block, step, and jab. It is important to watch what your opponent will do with their body and hands when being jabbed at with a single or a double jab. Once in striking position, step and jab followed by striking with fast combinations mixing speed with power.
   See figure CV-2

3.  The **Muhammad Ali Jab** is for a striker with good footwork. You will move side to side and in and out while jabbing an opponent. This allows you to control the pace and movement, setting your opponent up for single shots or combinations (mixing both hard and fast strikes).
    See figure CV-3

4.  The **Tommy Hearn's**, Ali, Sugar Ray Leonard Jab. This jab starts from a lower position close to the hip/waistline. The arm is in a V-shape with the fist on the inside hip to begin with and then coming straight up (holding the V-shape) striking the head, arms, and hands. As you observe how your opponent is reacting to this jab; be at the ready to counter with a straight power punch to the head or body. If your opponent throws a power punch, slip and counter with a power punch of your own (be set!). See figures CV-4 & CV-5

5.  The **Sugar Ray,** Larry Holmes, Hearns, Ali jab. This is a straight jab to the inside lower body. You will position your body away from your opponent and strike with a long lower jab to the stomach, making sure your shoulder is protecting your chin. Be aware that a counter right or left is in order in-case your opponent tries one of his own.
    See figure CV-6

6.  The **Hearns Fade/Gauge Jab**. This jab is a knock-off from the old right-cross in that it temporally blinds your opponent. Jab a few times utilizing the many jabs described above. Eventually position yourself close enough to your opponent to place the jab in their eyes for a split second, temporarily blinding them, and then strike with a powerful straight shot to the chin or body. If you can't see their eyes when the jab is positioned, they can't see yours. That is when you strike. This can also be called a gauge jab if not intended for the eyes but rather just the head or body. See figure CV-7

7.  The **Mike Tyson Jab**. This is my favorite because of its power and control. Once you can get in the soft or hard position utilizing your defenses or offenses, this jab is a powerful straight strike just like a straight right only it's a stiff straight left. Position your chin over your knee and strike putting your knee, hip, and shoulder into the punch for maximum power and control. You can also step in or just let your opponent run into it by timing their forward movement.
    See figure CV-8

**Another thing to practice is; jabbing straight outside and away from the head (towards the ear) drawing the head out knowing it will come back in. When it does, have that power punch ready. You can even straight jab towards the opposite ear drawing the head in towards a solid punch.**

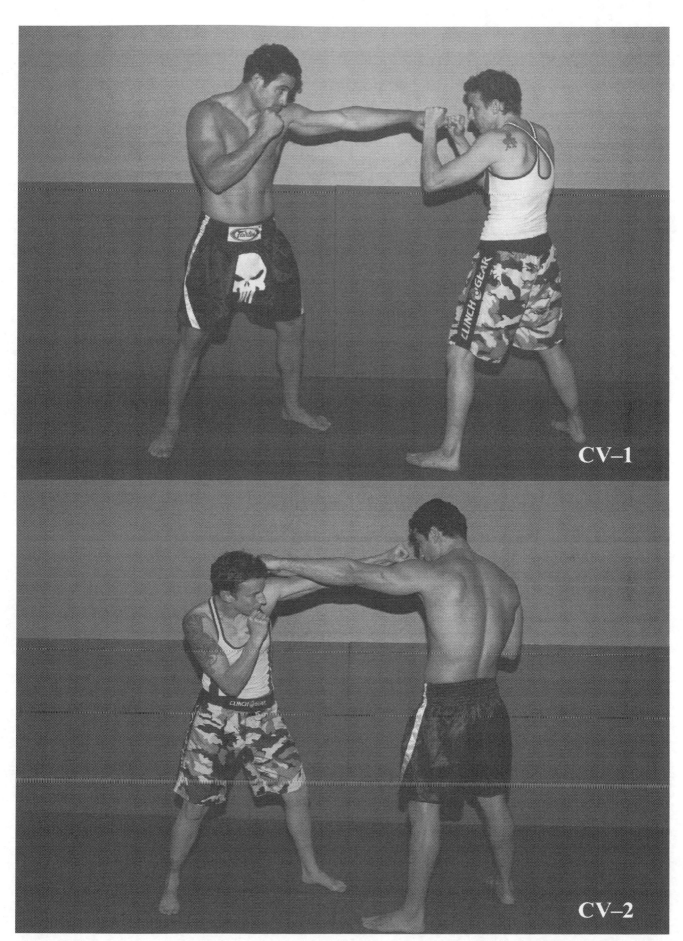

CV–1

CV–2

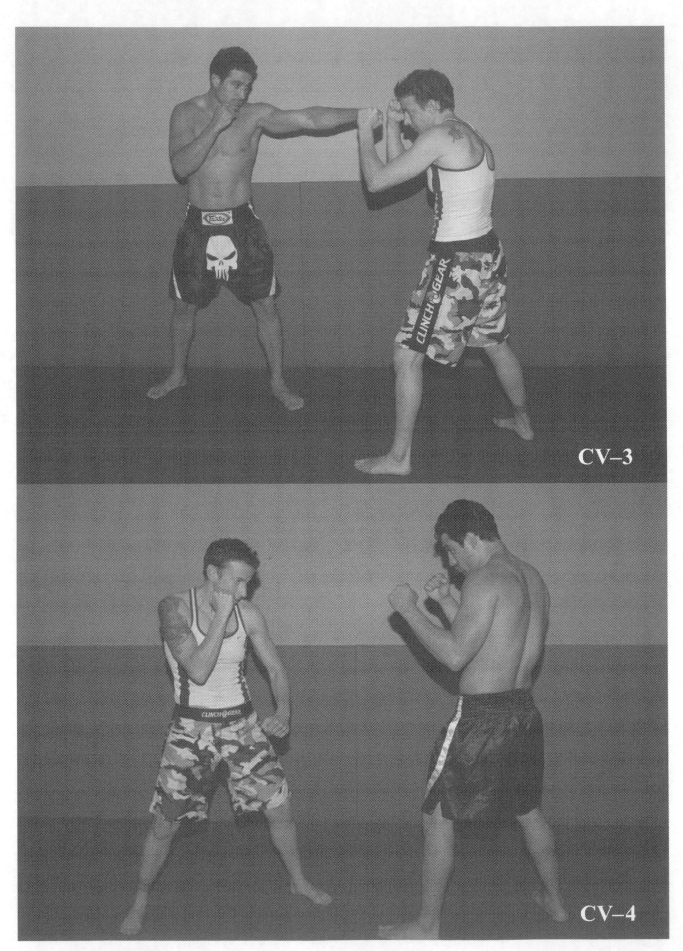

CV–3

CV–4

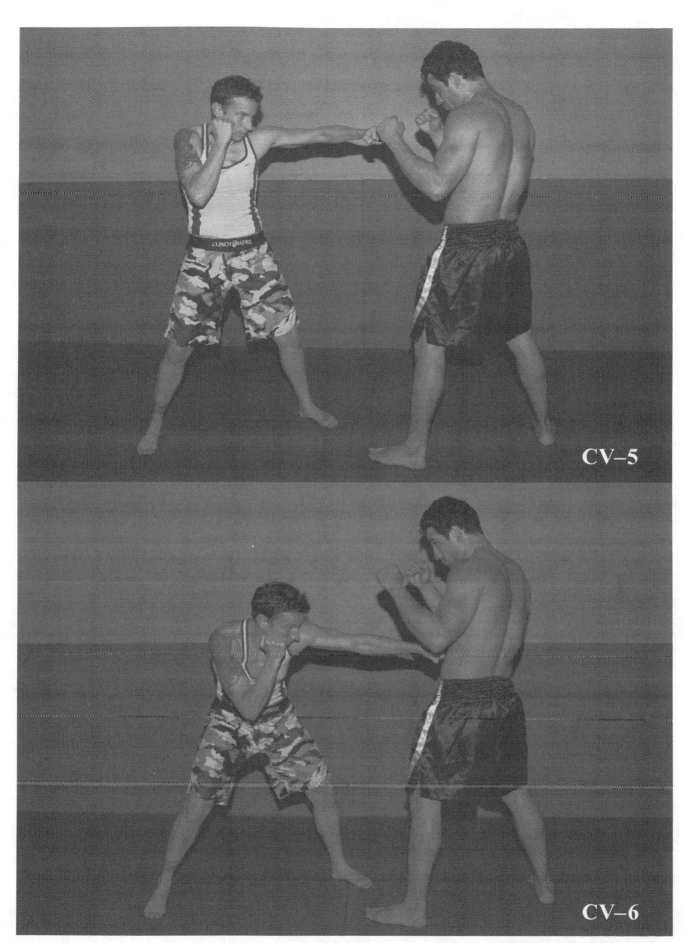

CV–5

CV–6

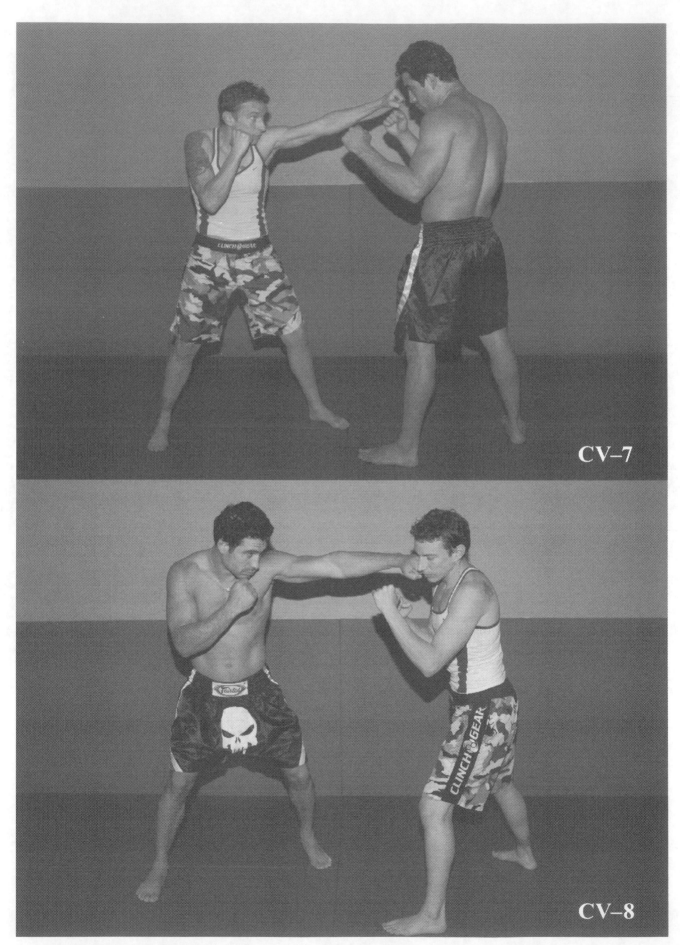

CV–7

CV–8

## Lefts and Rights

### Introduction

The lefts and rights we are going to cover are thrown from the long, medium, and close ranges. They are aimed at weak, soft, or guarded parts of an opponent's body or head. As a matter of fact, lefts and rights are thrown at the whole body from many different directions and speeds. Like a game of chess, you use the jabs as pawns and run the other chess pieces towards your opponent to beat them down and out as quickly and efficiently as possible with out harming yourself.

- The **Outside Left hook** is commonly used by most fighters and is brought to the opponent from outside the body and around the opponents guard and to the weak parts of the head or guard.
  See figures CV-9 & CV-10

- The **Inside Left hook** comes from inside the body and directly to the opponents head or guard.
  See figures CV-11 & CV-12

- The **Left Uppercut** can be from the inside or outside and will be directed under the chin or arm.
  See figures CV-13 & CV-14

- The **Upperhook** or **"Sweep"** is between an inside hook and an outside uppercut. The upper hook utilizes the "shift weight and come back" or the "shift weight and follow through" method of attack mentioned in the Power Punching section later in the book.
  See figures CV-15 thru CV-17

- The **Left Elbow** is from the close position and can be an upper elbow, a hook elbow, a jam elbow, or a downward elbow for MMA striking purposes.
  See figures CV-18 thru CV-20

- The **Outside Right Hook** is commonly used by most fighters and is brought to the opponent from an outside the body and around the opponents guard and to the weak parts of the head or directly at the guard.
  See figures CV-21

- The **Inside Right Hook** is coming from inside the body and directly to the opponents head or guard.
  See figures CV-22

- The **Overhand Right** is thrown like a military man would throw a hand grenade. This strike lands on the weak parts of the head.
  See figures CV-23

- The **Fast Straight Right** is from the inside and is just that, fast! With the speed; will come power.
  See figure CV-24

- The **Hard Straight Right** is just that, coming to your opponent with all you got!
  See figure CV-25

- The **Right Uppercut** can be from the inside or outside and will be directed under the chin or arms.
  See figures CV-26

- The **Right Upperhook or "Sweep"** is between an inside hook and an outside uppercut. This utilizes the "shift weight and come back" or the "shift weight and follow through" method of attack mentioned in the Power Punching section later in the book.
  See figures CV-27 thru CV-30

- The **Right Elbows** are from the close position and can be an upper elbow, a hook elbow, a jam elbow, or a downward elbow for MMA striking purposes.
  See figures CV-31 thru CV-35

## Fast Punches versus Hard Punches

All of the strikes mentioned above can be utilized with either fast or hard delivery. The **fast strike** mainly utilizes the arm and shoulder.
See figure CV-36

The **hard strike** is also fast except that you will be putting you toes, knee, and hip into the strike. The toe, knee, hip, movement resembles and therefore is referred to as "Squashing the Bug". While in your boxing stance, the fist and forearm will go forward while at the same time rotating your toes inward which in turn will rotate your knee, which in turn will rotate your hip. With this motion, half of your body is moving towards your opponent's body with speed and force like no other. You will want to shock and awe your opponent's anatomy sending them reeling in pain or putting them to sleep.
See figure CV-37

## Feinting

## Introduction

## "The Judicious Feint"

There is not a single boxer in the land that does not appreciate the great value of a judicious feint. The practice of feinting a blow in order to draw an opponent off their guard, leaving an opening to attract them into a nice lead or to disguise the nature of an intended lead, is of universal usage. Every able boxer should place it close to the top of their list of accomplishments.

Bear in mind that you can not be indecisive. Make up your mind quickly and start right in to suit the action to the thought. The best times to capitalize on feints are when your opponent is nervous, as in the first round, when they are hurt, or tired. Feinting is generally called into play before straight leads to the head or body, the left hand being the most frequently employed. Practice the feints a few times on your opponent to see what they do. Do they cover up? Do they drop their hands? Do they flinch?

When it is desired, send a right or left to the face, feinting low with the left as though to land to the ribs or lower body. The opponent will naturally seek to block this blow and in doing so will be compelled to bring down all or part of their guard, leaving their face more or less exposed for an attack. At the same time you must remember to guard your own face with the free hand.

When contemplating a lead for the body, feint to the face, thus drawing your opponent's guard high. Guard yourself and send in the blow in the manner described in the preceding sentence.

- The **Leg** feint consists of stepping forward with the lead foot only, as if trying to get into your mid to close position. Then step back into the long position and fire a long straight shot at the head. You can also utilize a short jab with this arm feint making it a **jab and leg** feint. Practice going for the upper and lower body, keeping your opponent constantly guessing as to what is coming next.

- The **Arm** feint is achieved with the arm partially straightened making a forward movement of the hand. Strike as if you are aiming for the face but stopping just short of it and bam! A straight right follows directly behind it either to the head or body. You can integrate your footwork into the feints as well, moving to the side, feinting, and then letting the shot go.

- The **Shoulder** feint often accompanies the arm feint. Simply bring your shoulder forward, accompanied by a slight forward movement of the arm or hand.

- The **Head** feint is another advantage you have at your disposal. Simply yet swiftly move/ bend your head forward, then back, and then strike.

- The **kick** feint is great for drawing your opponent's body lower. Shift your right hip and knee forward as if going for a low or mid kick positioning your chin over your opposite knee. Fire off a nice stiff left or right to the chin or body.

- The **Eye** feint is underutilized. Use your eyes to draw an opponent down or to a particular position by looking towards their body feinting down and hitting up. To go to the body do the opposite. Look at their head, feint towards their head, and then go to the body.

The successful feinter invariably uses considerable footwork, stepping forward, backward, to the right or to the left, keeping their arms in motion. Always stay balanced for a quick recovery. Practice the combination feints to keep your opponents guessing at all times.

Summed up, feinting is one of the prettiest, most spectacular, and at the same time extremely effective attributes of boxing. This is especially true when used in conjunction with your defense and counter punching.

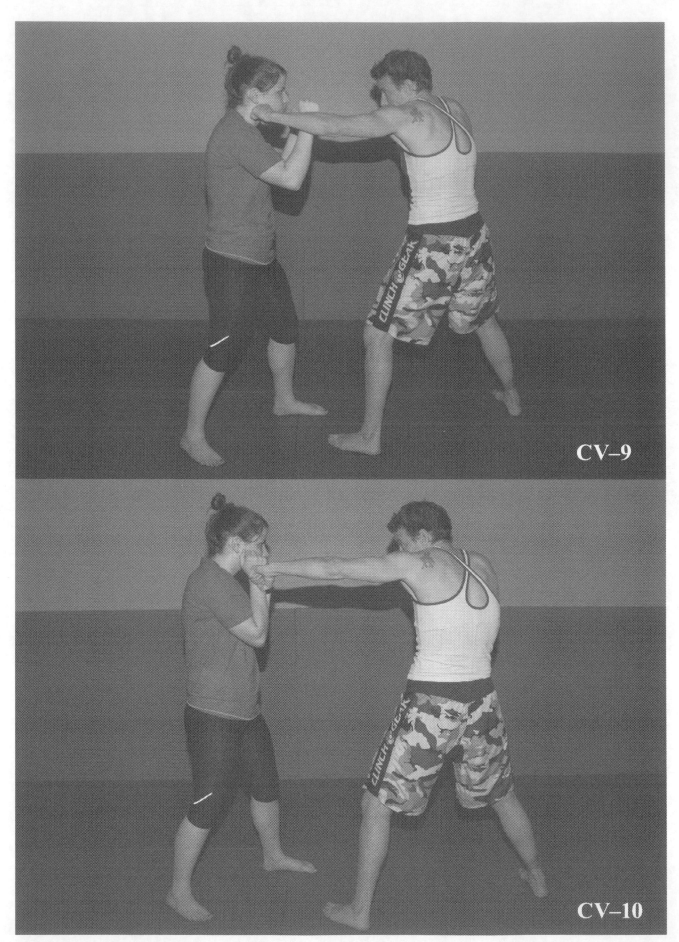

CV–9

CV–10

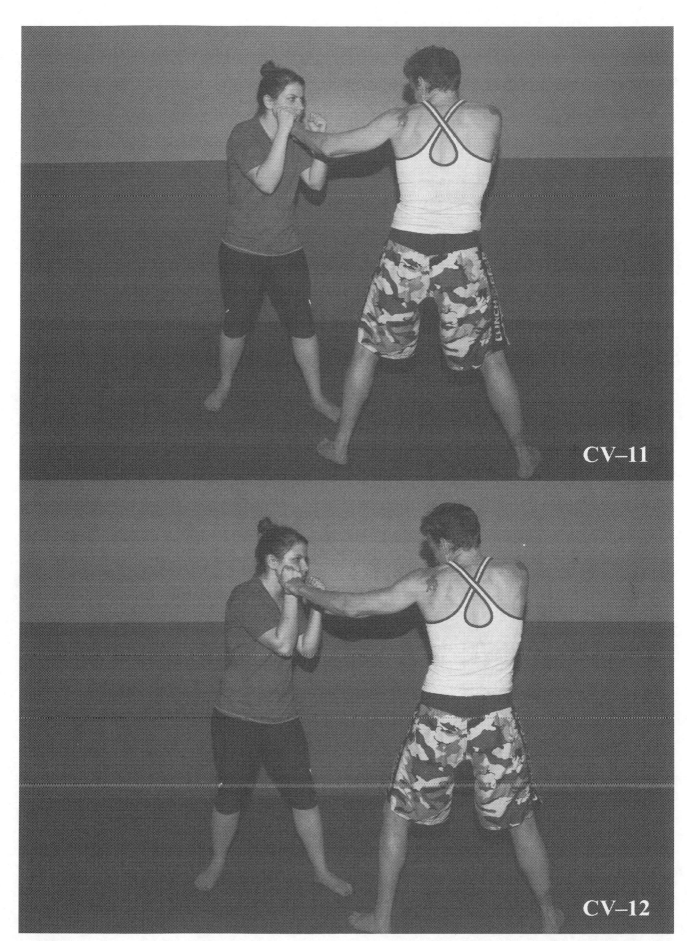

CV–11

CV–12

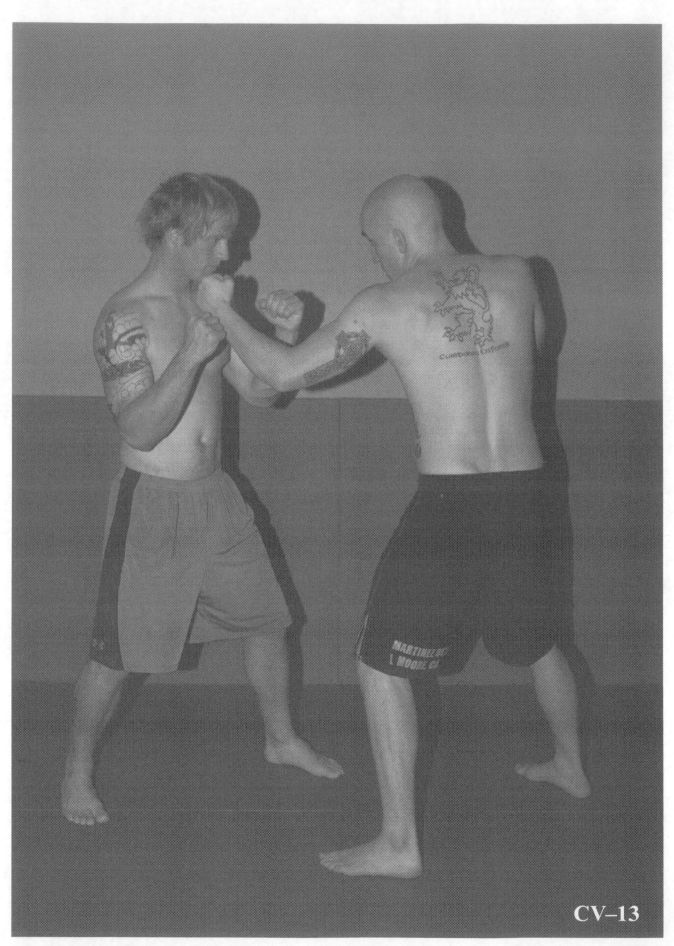

CV–13

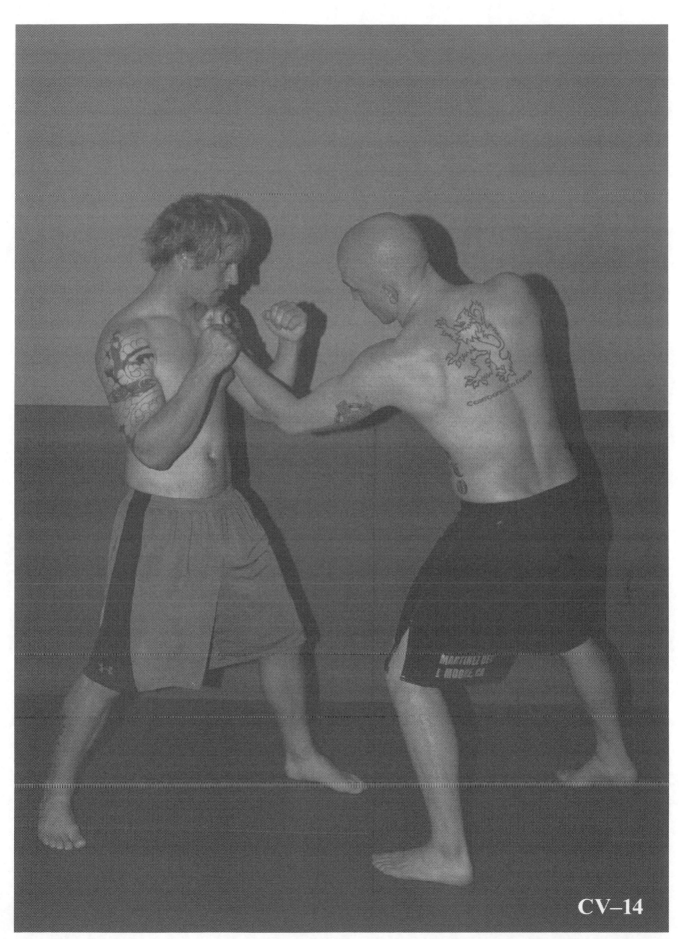

CV–14

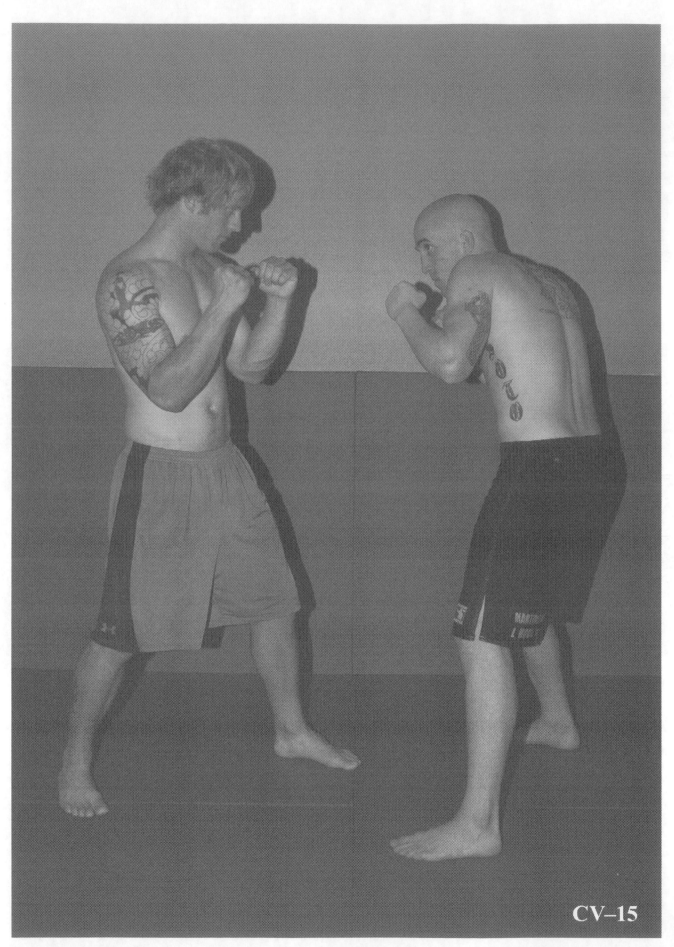

CV–15

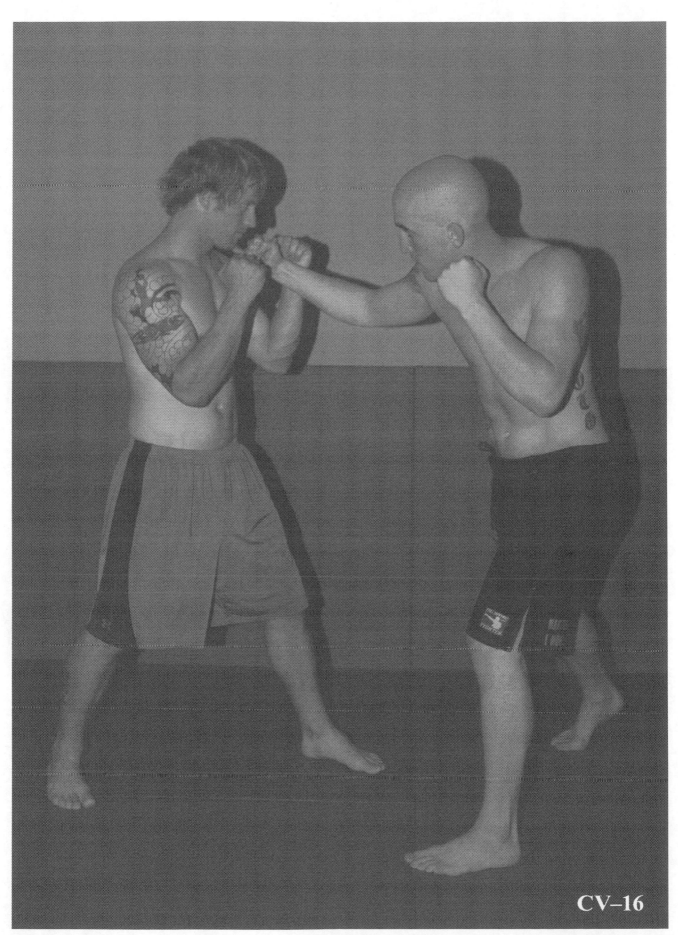

CV–16

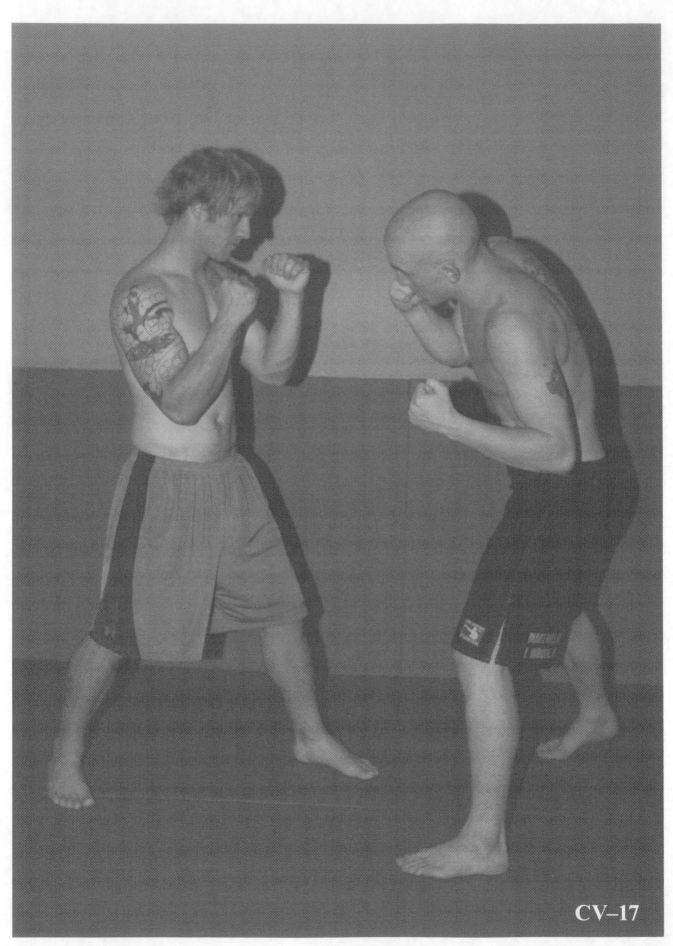

CV–17

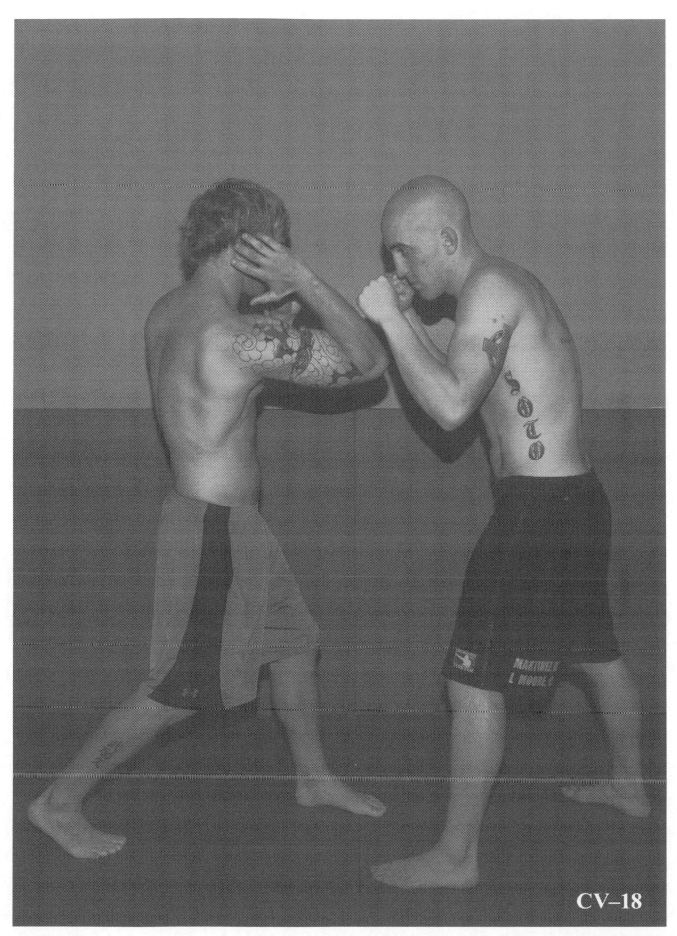

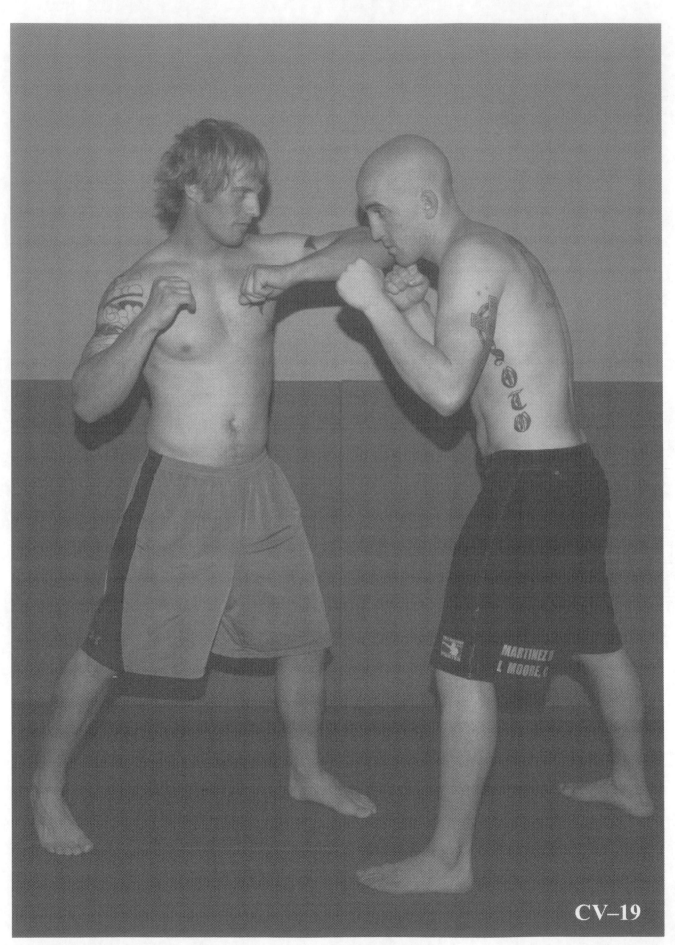

CV–19

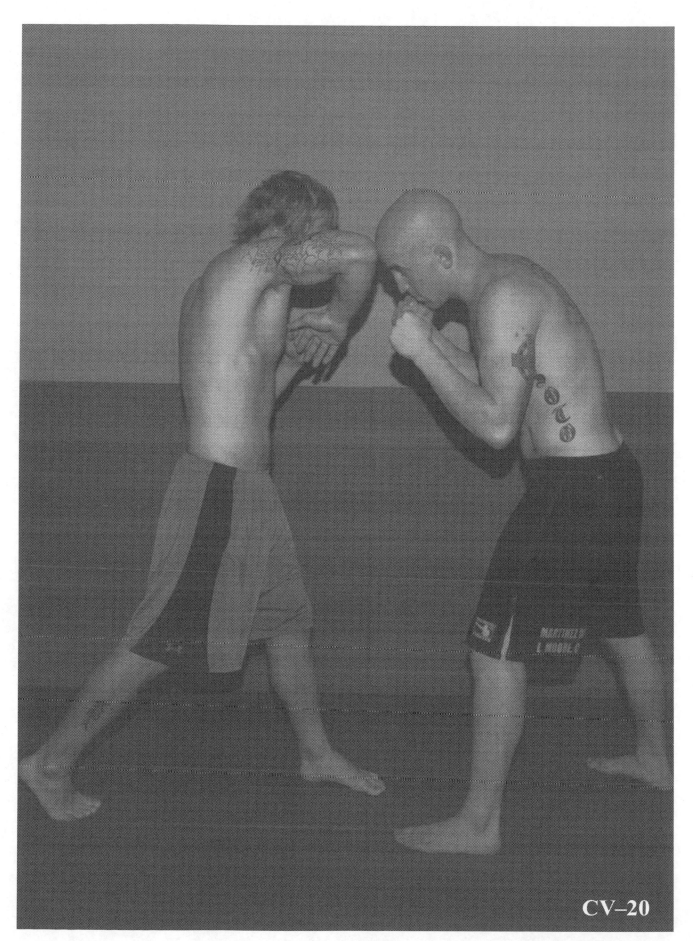

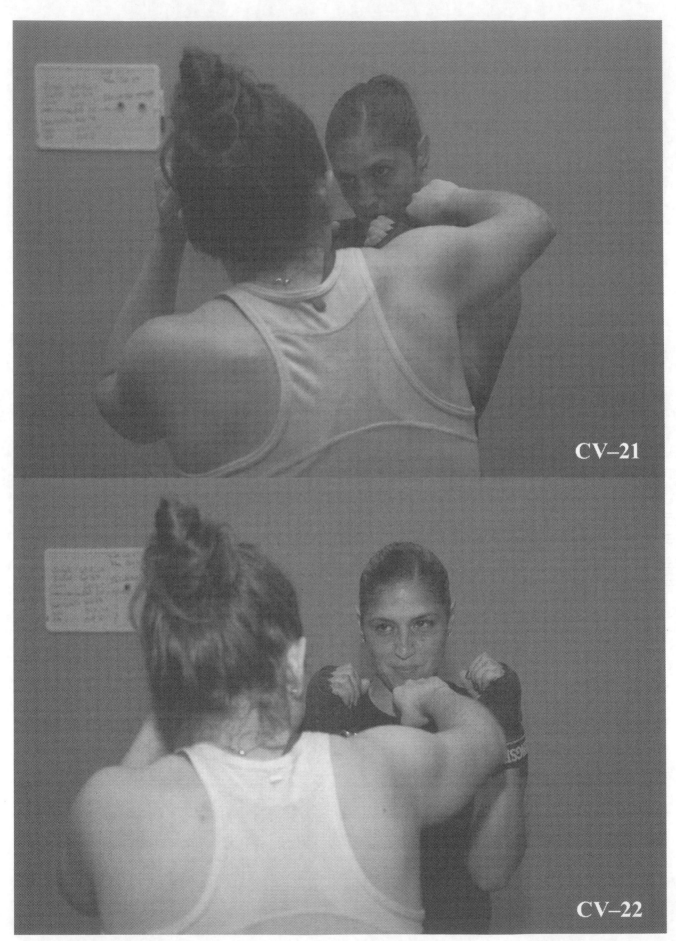

CV–21

CV–22

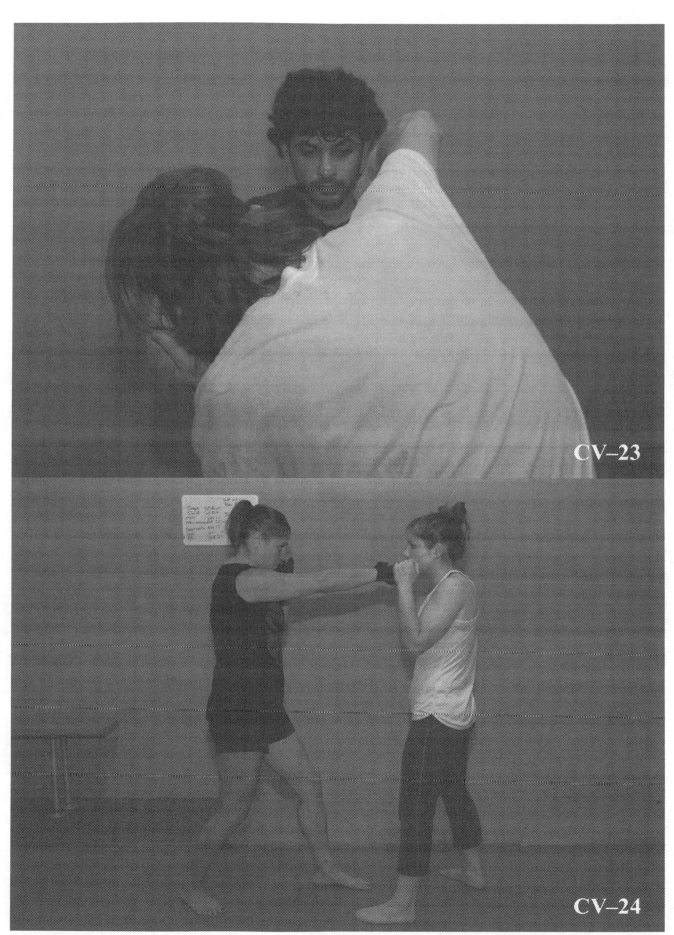

CV–23

CV–24

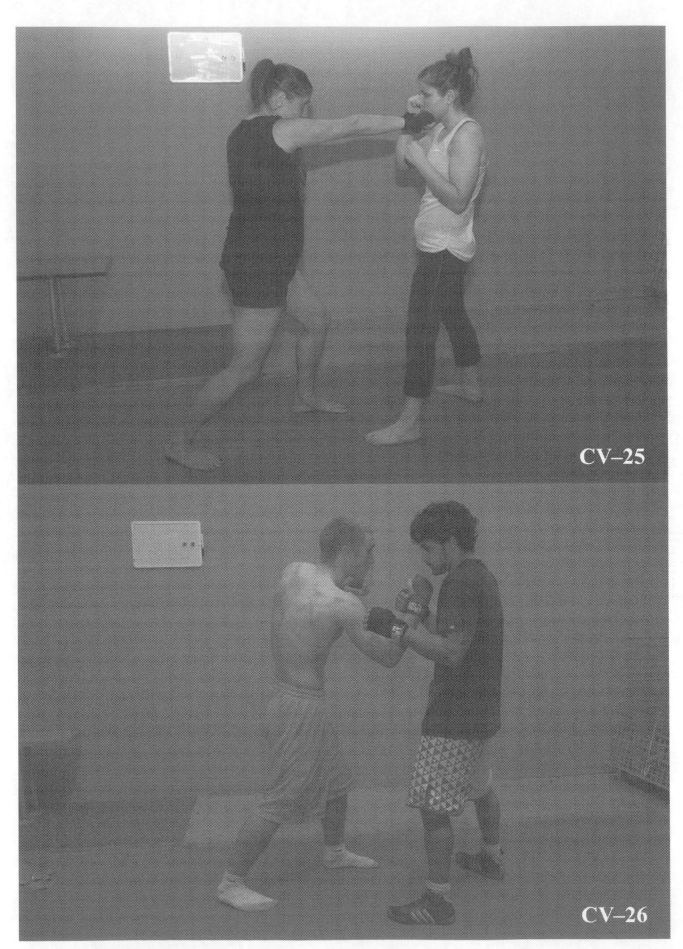

CV–25

CV–26

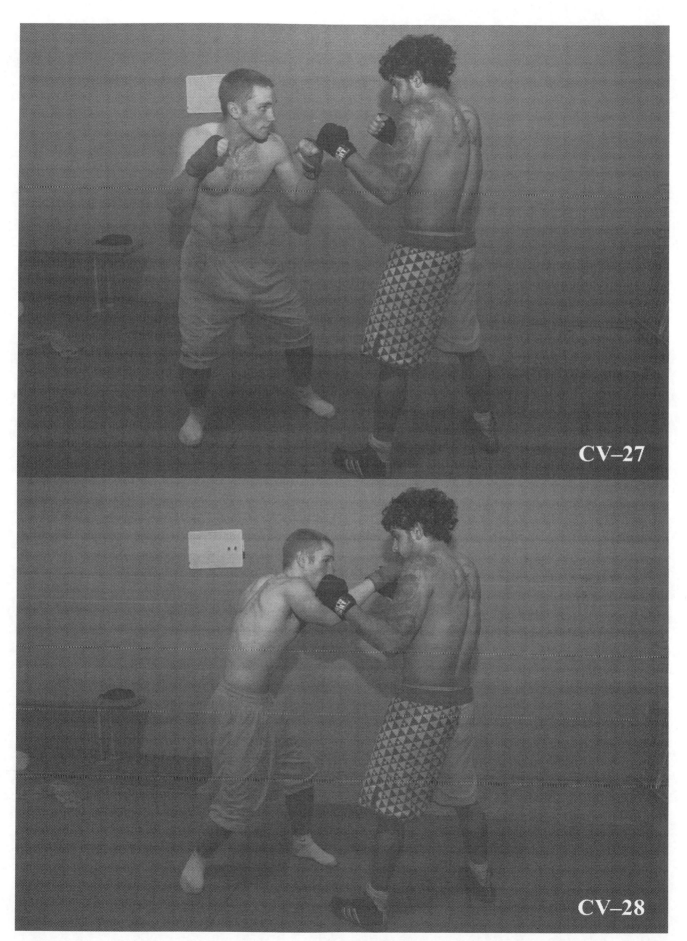

CV–27

CV–28

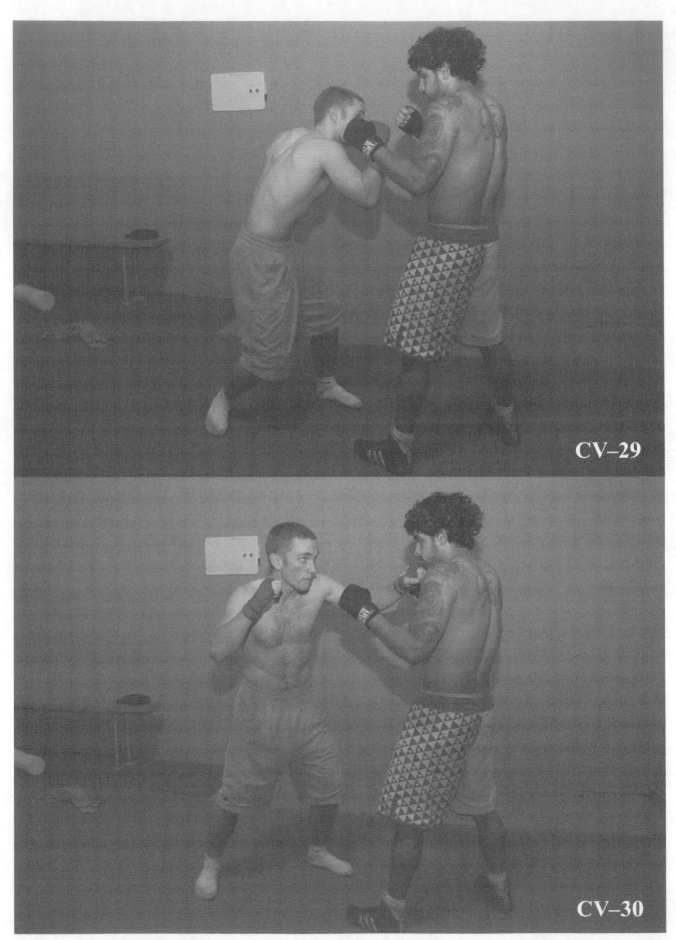

CV–29

CV–30

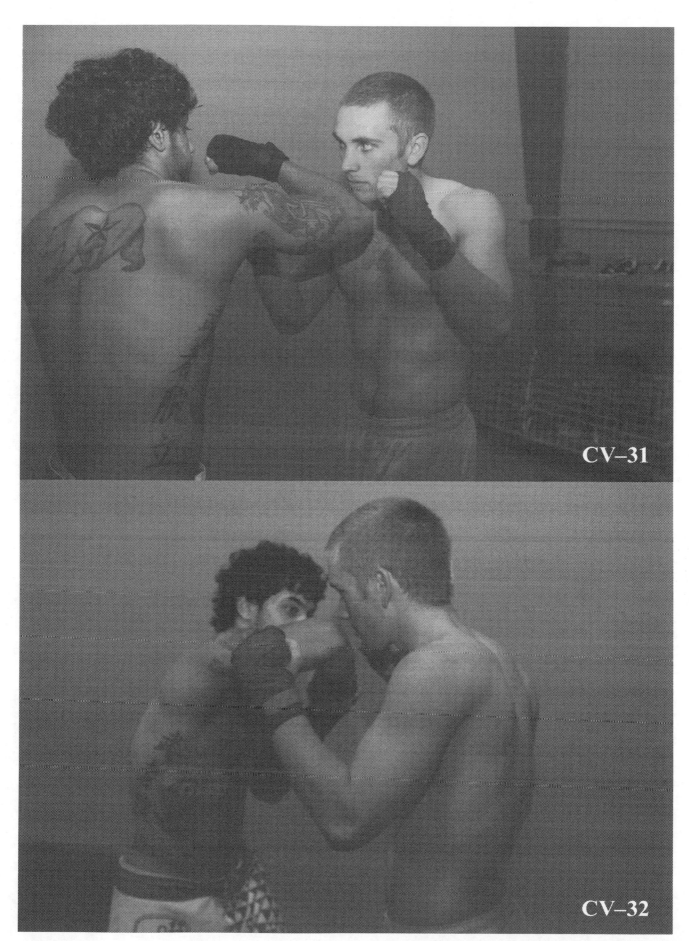

CV–31

CV–32

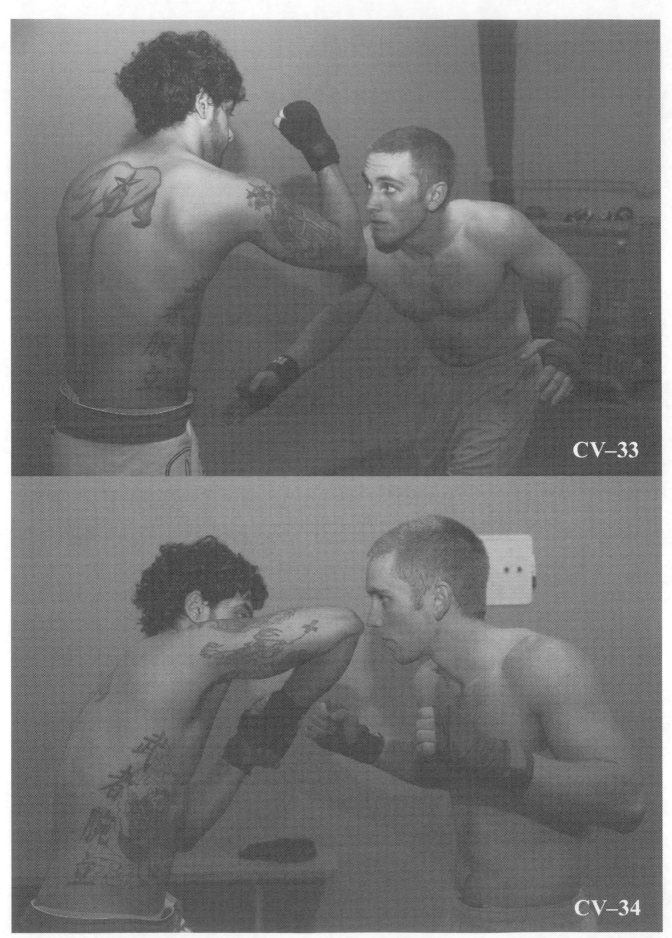

CV–33

CV–34

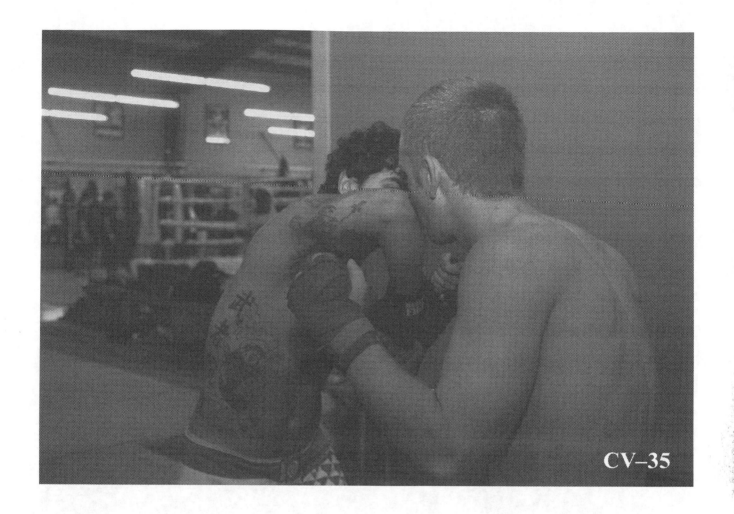

CV–35

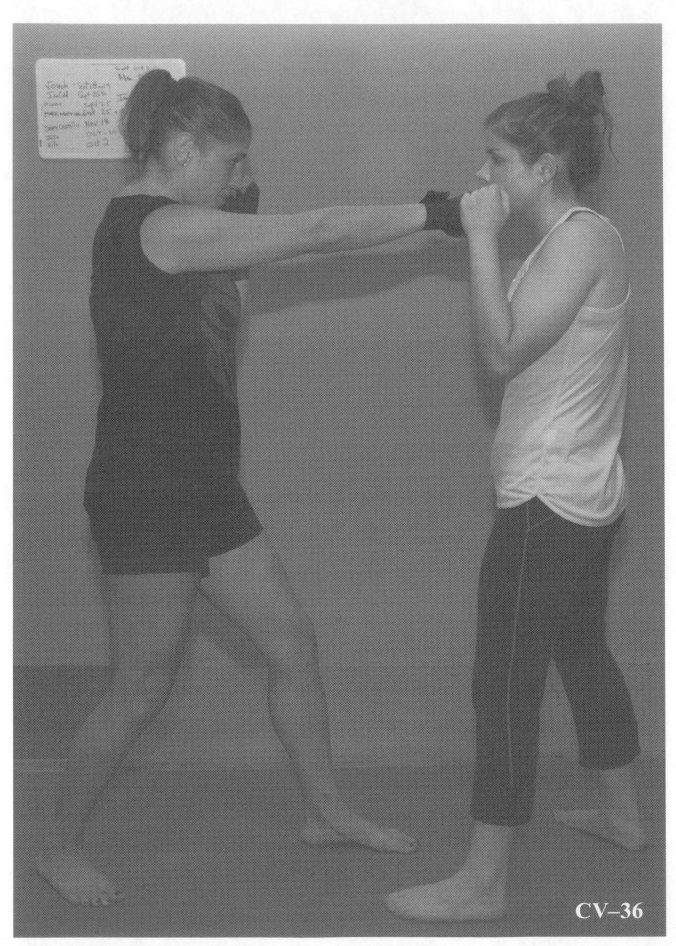

CV–36

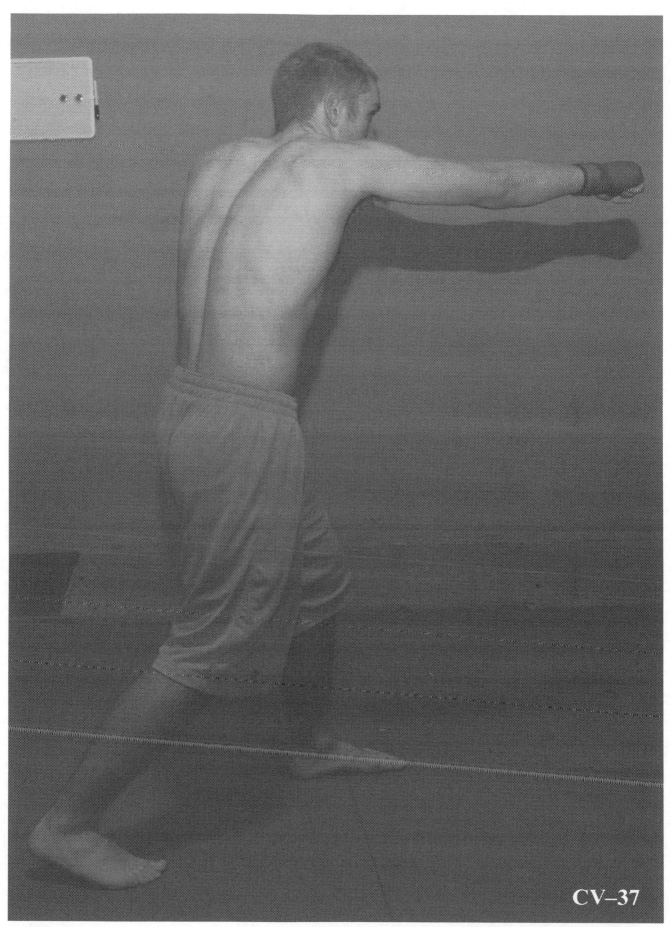

CV–37

## Breathing

### Introduction

I cannot stress enough the necessity of proper **breathing technique** during a bout. You must practice breathing while exercising and training in order to get the most out of yourself. With proper breathing alone you can add many more rounds to your workout. This in turn will enable you to learn and do more than the opponent that faces you across the cage or ring. It is sad but true that the majority of athletes do not know how to breathe. Like all other sports, strikers and boxers should place a special importance on this vital point.

**Control** your breathing throughout the workout as mentioned in Chapter III Defenses. Exhale (breathe) through your nose as you are punching. You can exhale through your mouth but be sure to keep your jaw closed. Do not hold your breathe when throwing single or combinations of punches.

In between strikes, control your breathing by relaxing and slowing your breathing down. If you are tired and need more time, get away from your opponents striking distance and take a deep breath. If you get winded, you can get your wind back and stay in control by utilizing your defenses and staying cool, calm, and relaxed. Avoid becoming anxious and out of control as this will cause you to lose your rhythm and poise leaving yourself open to unwanted punishment.

At the end of each round take deep breaths. Fill your lungs up and let it out slowly. Breathe down into your lower stomach thus lowering your heart rate and clearing your head. Your head and mind can become fuzzy when your body is tired, compromising your ability to take a hit and increasing the likelihood of getting hurt.

## Power Punching

### Introduction

**Power Punching or Knockout Blows** are what we as spectators and combatants live to see and do. Strikers and Boxers alike strive to accomplish that one hard blow to the body or head that will cause their opponent to crumble to their force. (As mentioned earlier about former boxing champions that had that punch and power.) Currently, up and coming MMA strikers are getting their due behind their knockout power punches.

A "knockout" is a punch or blow that renders an opponent unable to continue for ten seconds or more. It can be delivered in various ways to different points of the body and head. The good thing about MMA fighters is that there are no standing eight counts as there are in boxing. All you have to do is hurt your opponent for a few seconds and the referee will stop the bout.

To get the most out of your power punches you must utilize the "Squash the Bug" method. This requires turning your toes into the punch, which in turn will direct you knee into the punch, which in turn will get your hip involved thereby creating the knockout punch. If it's a hard right punch, than it will be your right toes that lead the party. If it's your left, than it will be your left toes that lead the attack.
See figure CV-37

You can power punch from the regular guard by having your head and body centered. You can also do this from the hard position which is having your chin over either of your knees.

- One way to power punch is to **shift your weight and come back.** You can accomplish this in the regular guard or from the hard position. Strike (explode) with power and control to the weak part of your opponent's anatomy then quickly return to your original position. You are looking to shock and awe your opponent as well as the crowd.
See figures CV-38 thru CV-40

- The other way to power punch is to **shift your weight and follow through.** This punch is by way of the hard position. Explode your weight and punch towards your opponent, following through with your head over your opposite knee. Then, shift back towards the other side, punching with exploding force, positioning your head over the opposite knee. Repeat this until the opponent is done. Shock and awe is what this is all about! See figures CV-41 thru CV-44

These power punches will be more effective when you direct those strikes at the pre-identified weak areas mentioned earlier in chapter IV "Strike Zones".
See figures CV-45 & CV-46

**Body Shots**

**Introduction**

The **Solar Plexus punch** or **body shot**, when delivered correctly, has a telling effect on an opponent. This shot is usually dealt in close quarters, since the advantage is greater. Socking the weak/soft parts of the body, as explained earlier, will make the body shot more effective while doing less damage to your hands than beating on an opponents head.

- Most fighters have a **3 –count body shot**, they:

    a. Get their position for the body shot

    b. Drop their preferred hand for the body shot,

    c. Strike at the body.
    See figures CV-47 thru CV-49

- I believe in the **2-count method**, since it has been proven on opponents through my past boxing experience.

    a. Lower your arm and hand into the perfect striking position at the same time you are moving into the lower striking zone. In other words, combine both 1 and 2 of the 3-count body shot above into a single movement.

b. Strike the soft (weak) parts of the body that were explained earlier in the Strike Zones Introduction Section. After the punch has been delivered, either stay there and keep punching or weave and step out.
See figures CV-50 & CV-51

Using feints to the head or a combination of defenses and offenses to the head will invariably open up the body shots on your opponent.

## In-Fighting (on or off the ropes)

## Introduction

**In-Fighting**, when done properly, can be very successful for you and very disappointing for your opponent. The main objective when in-fighting is to be able to hit your opponent without being hit. It is important to stay in an attack position leaving yourself able to defend or attack. When an opponent has you on the ropes, be sure to be in position to make them miss and make them pay, defensively and offensively. Do not have your back on the ropes or cage, rather just your butt for gauging and mobility. When you are on the ropes or cage have your shield up, legs set, and body low. Do not cover up as if you are scared to get hit! Stand ready, brave, and prepared for battle! This is where we separate the men from the boys!

- **The Shield:** Hands are up and engaged in constant movement to obtain an offensive position for some vicious body and head punching. Work the long-medium and medium-short range punches. You can use the offensive beat down and out strategy, the defense and counter movement, or both, enabling you to hit without getting hit or hurt.
  See figure CV-52

- **Long-medium range punches** are just that, long punches and leaning in for the medium punches (arm in V-shape).
  See figures CV-53 & CV-54

- **Medium-close range punches** are V-shape to L-shape arm positions.
  See figures CV-55 & CV-56

Be sure and work all defenses and offenses, then either:

1. Take one step out and position yourself to move back in to serve more punishment.

2. Stay there and utilize your defensive and/or offensive combinations to beat down your opponent until the referee stops the bout or the opponent is down and out.

3. Side step and/or pivot staying up close and personal.

4. Jab out or step and jab to either side or backwards.

When in the medium-short range, take one step back and fire off the hard one-two combination.

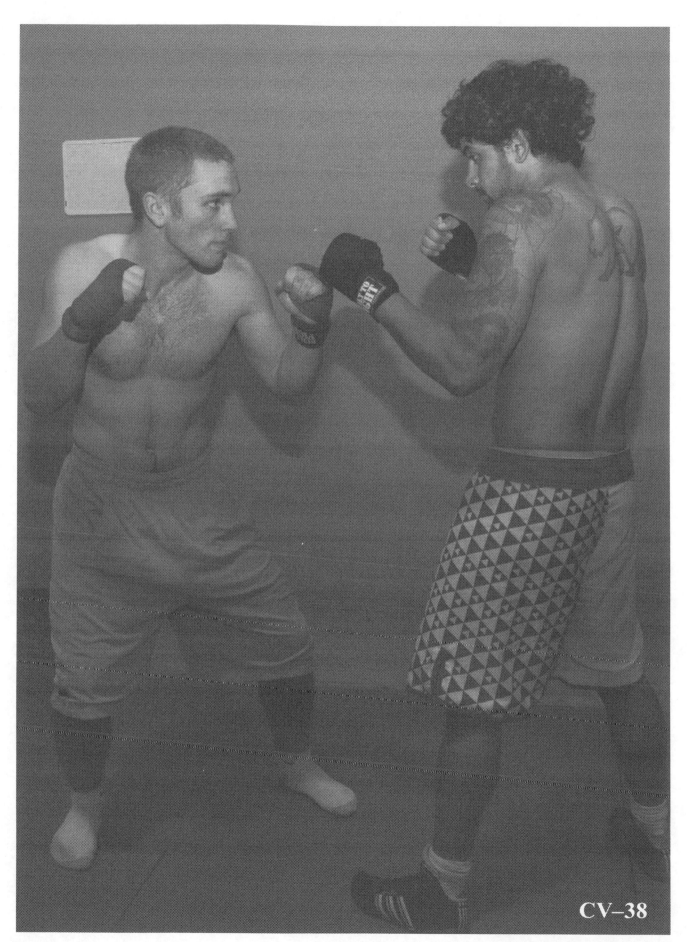

CV–38

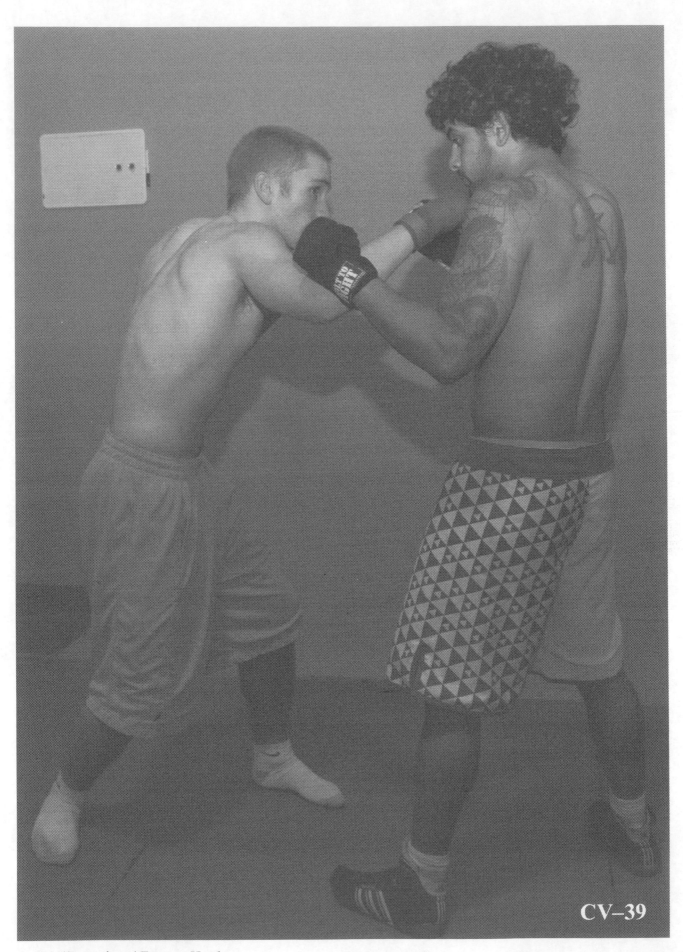

CV–39

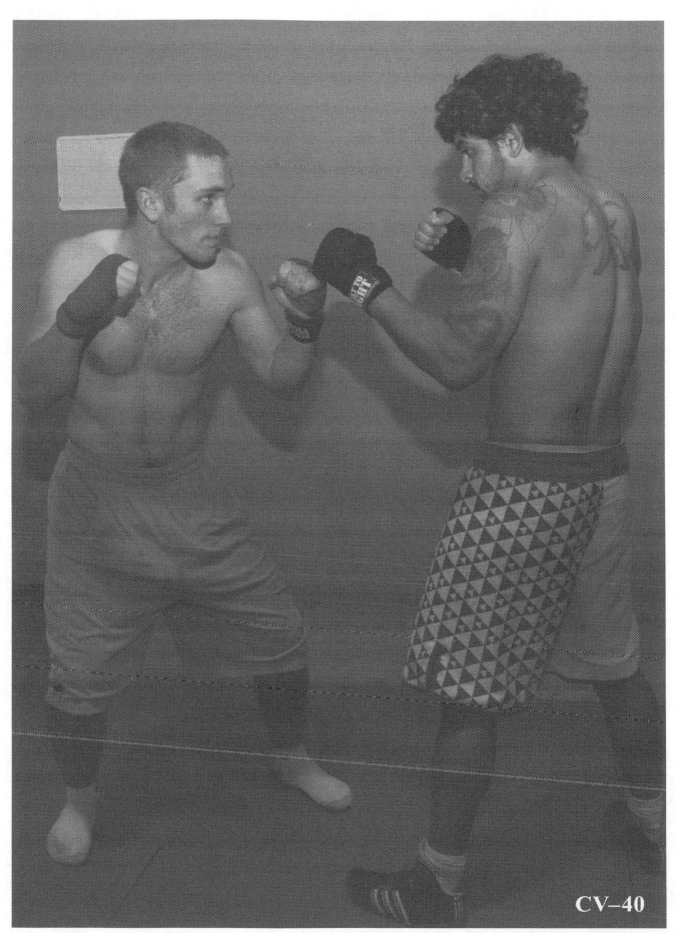

CV–40

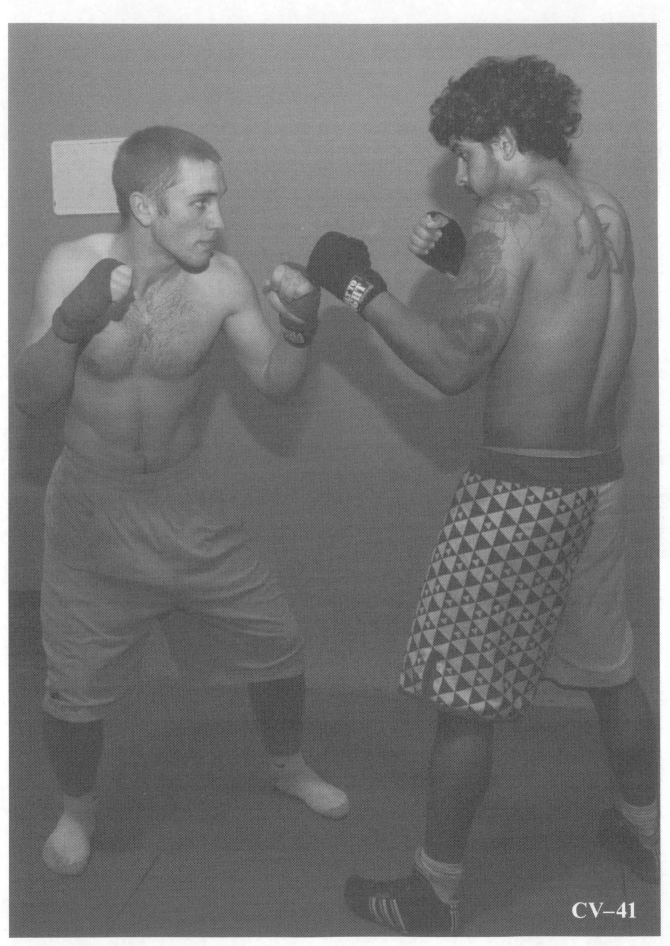

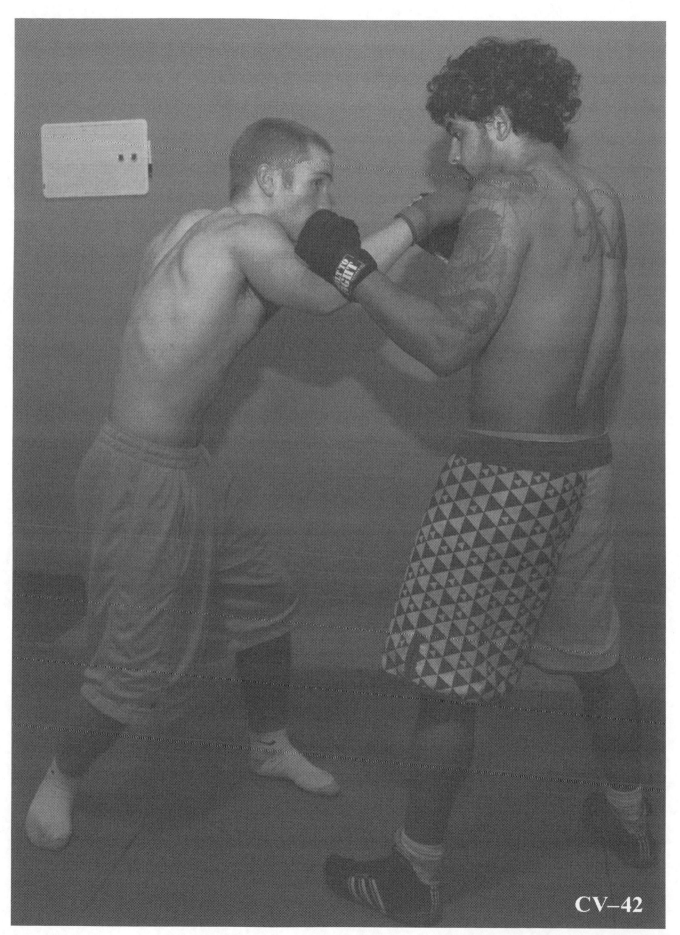

CV–42

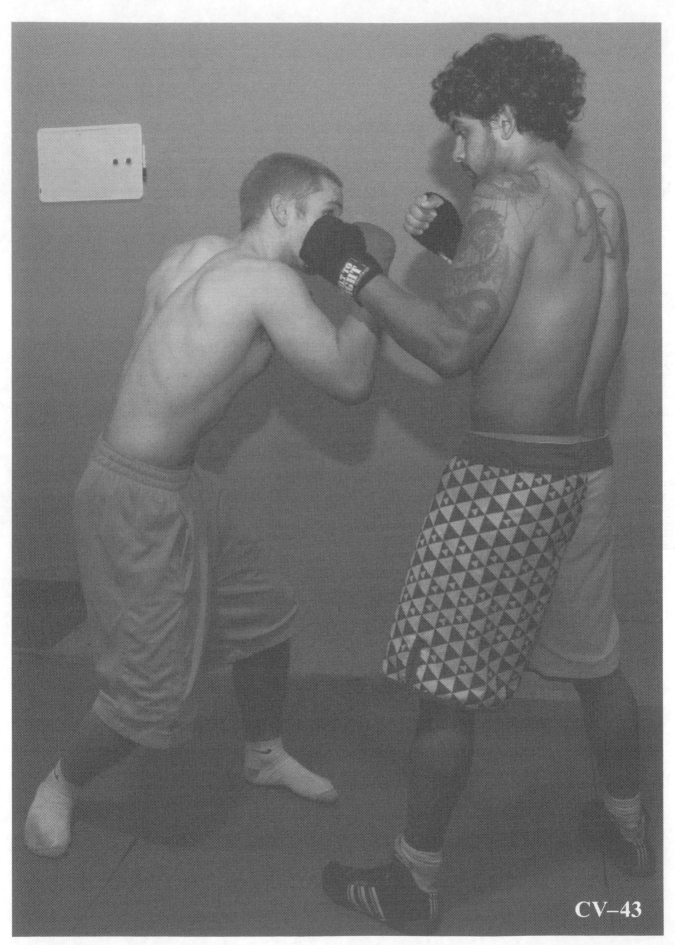

CV–43

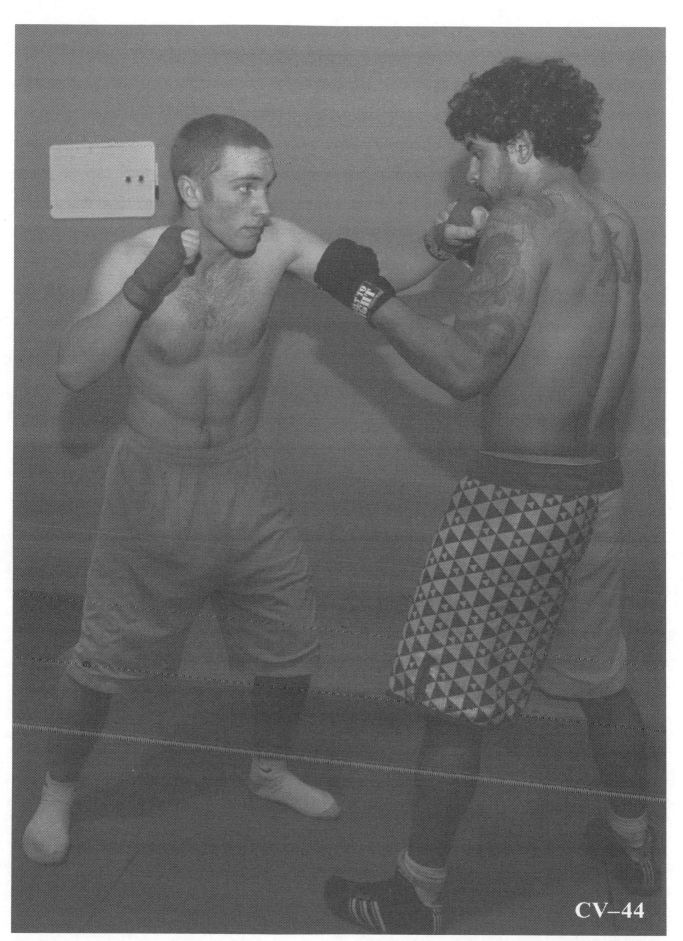

CV–44

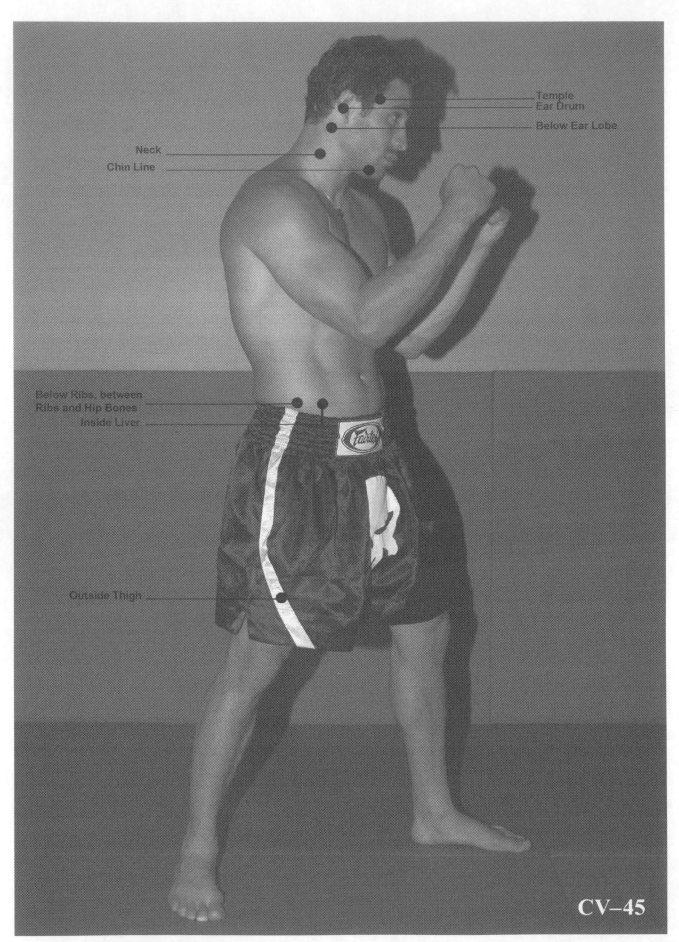

Temple
Ear Drum
Below Ear Lobe

Neck
Chin Line

Below Ribs, between
Ribs and Hip Bones
Inside Liver

Outside Thigh

**CV–45**

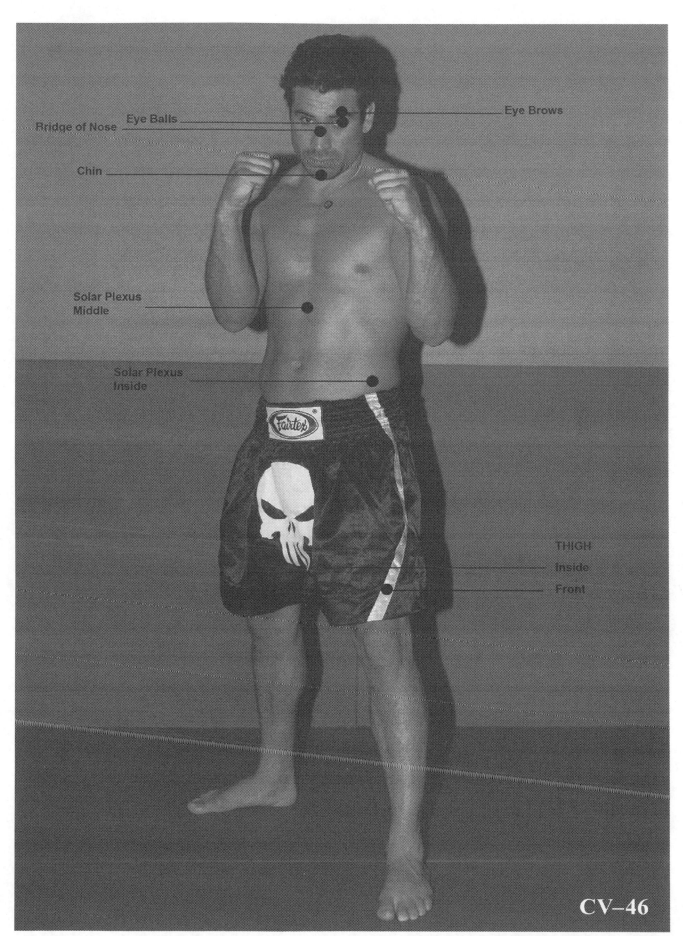

Bridge of Nose

Eye Balls

Eye Brows

Chin

Solar Plexus
Middle

Solar Plexus
Inside

THIGH

Inside

Front

CV–46

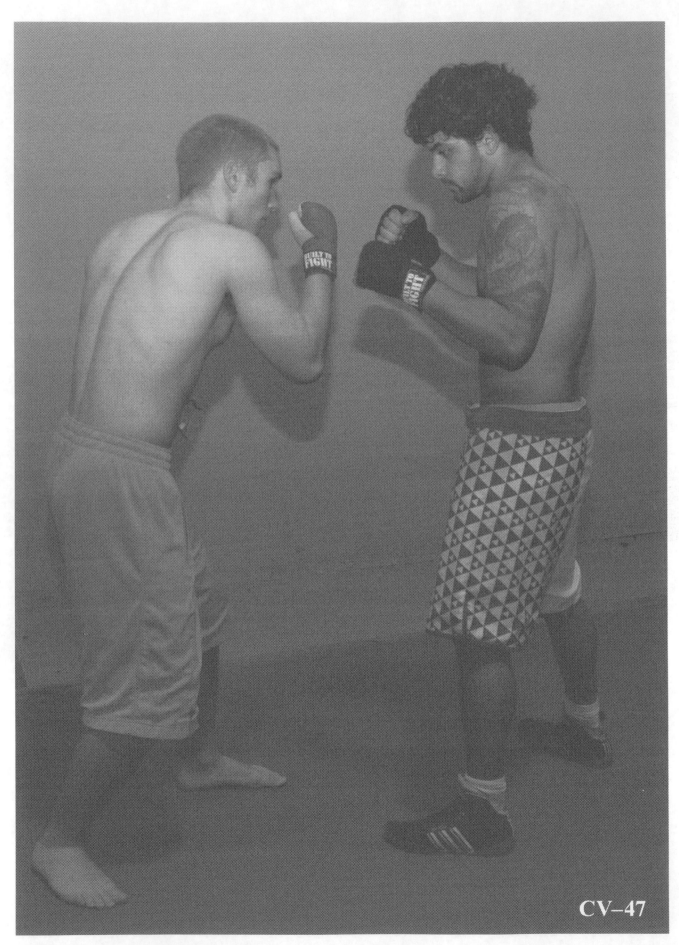

CV–47

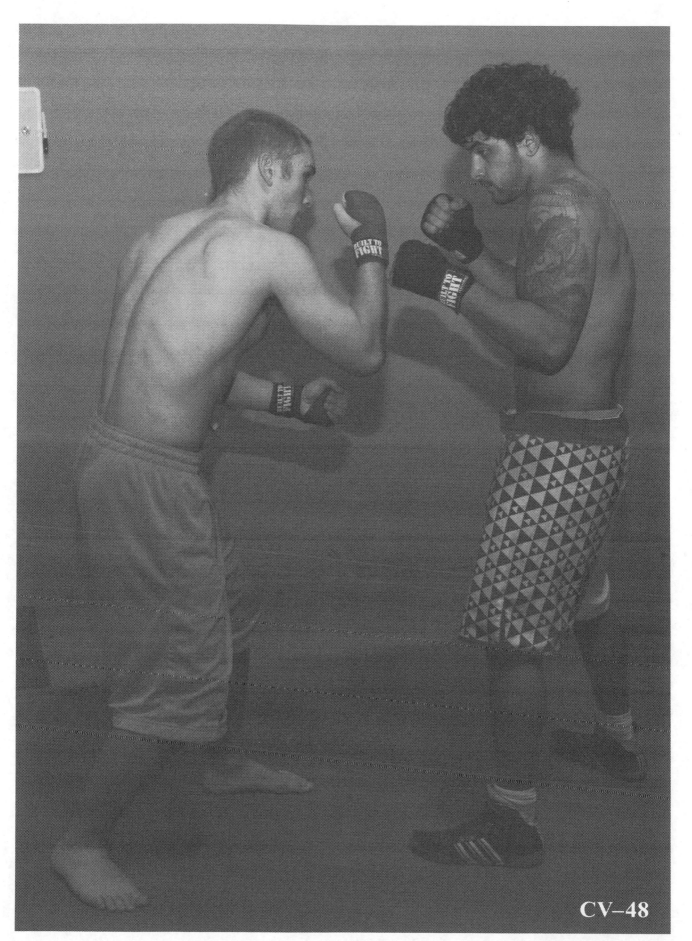

CV–48

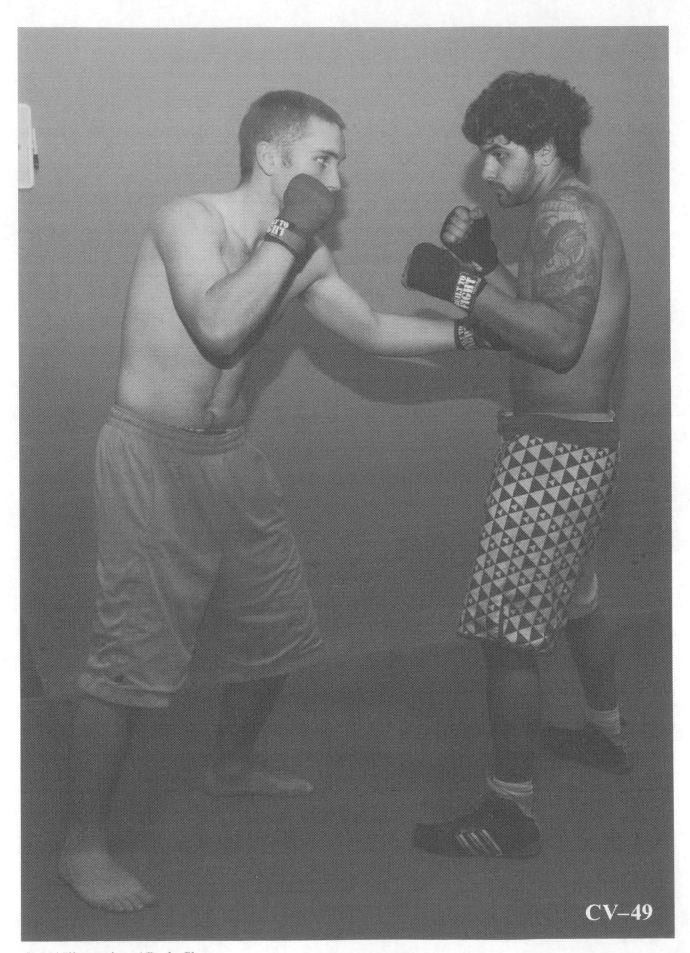

CV–49

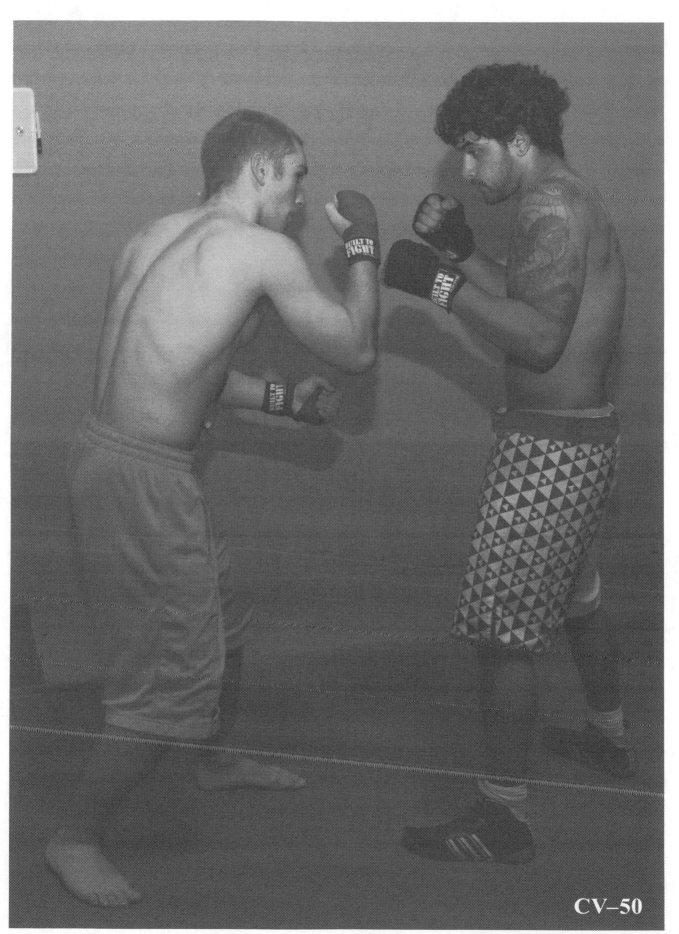

CV–50

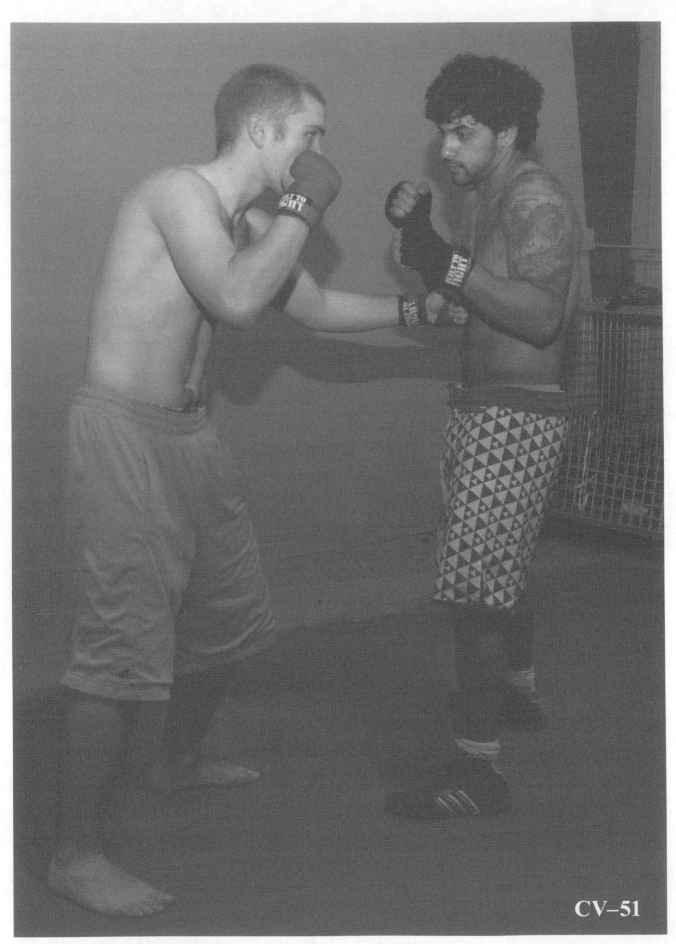

CV–51

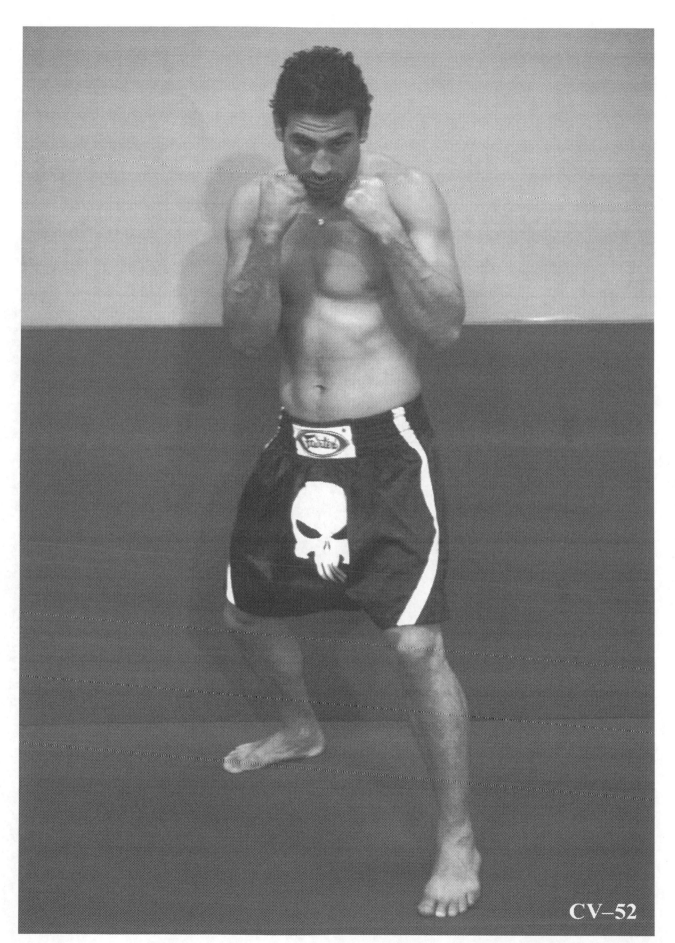

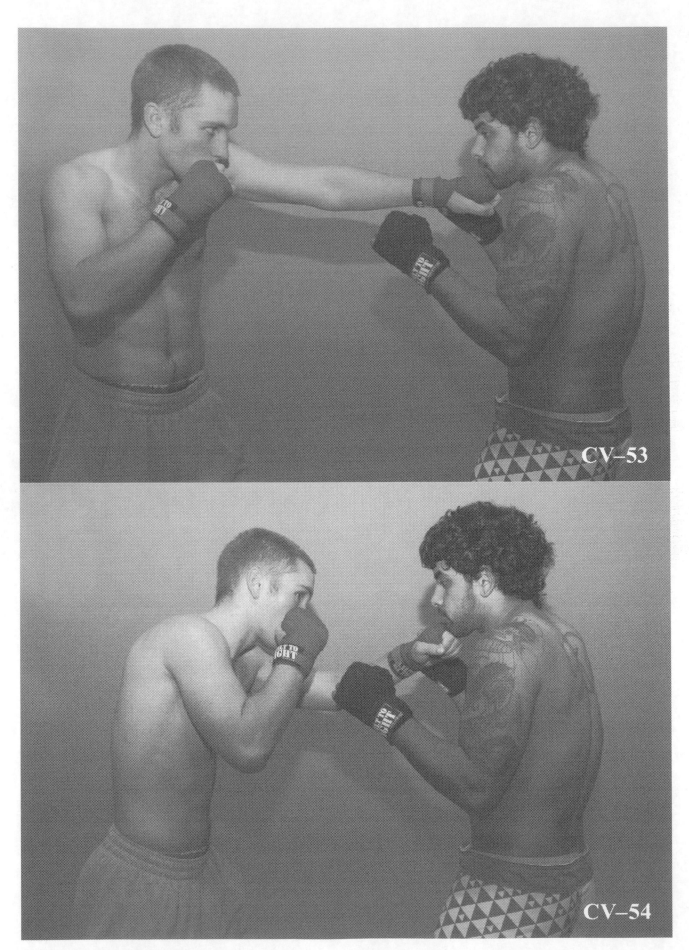

CV–53

CV–54

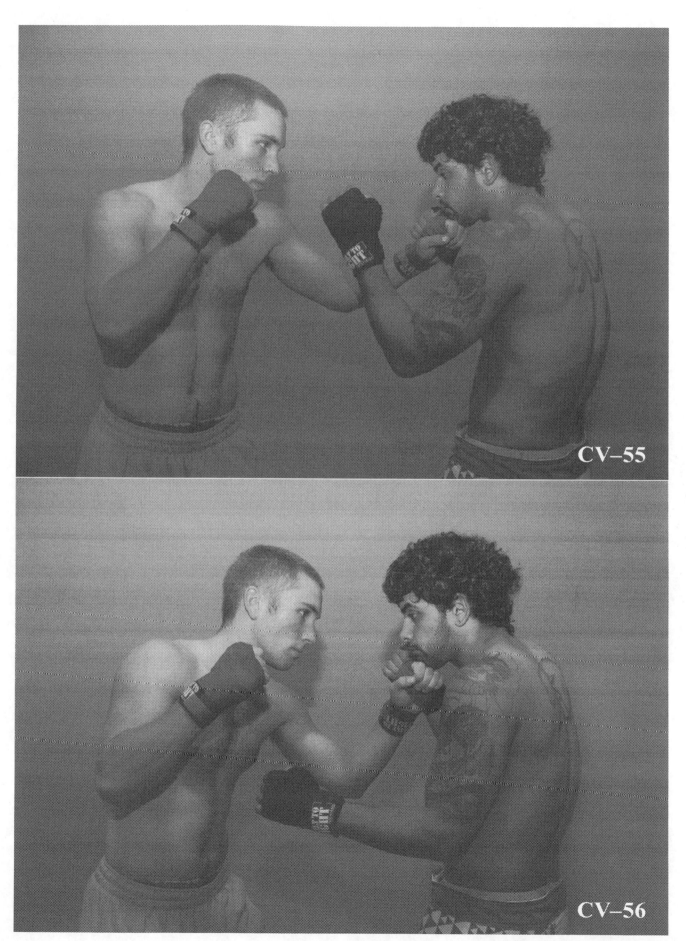

CV–55

CV–56

# **NOTES**

You'll want to let go of the power punches and counter punches at all times.  Practice utilizing the breathing techniques for better results.

## Shadow Boxing

### Introduction

**Shadow Boxing** is a very important feature in training.  When shadow boxing, go through the same motions as in actual competition.  Every movement utilized in actual competition can be practiced and developed through proper shadow boxing.  Shadow boxing develops speed, accuracy, breathing, endurance, positioning, and proper fighting technique.

Offense, defense, and all the little things that make a great champion are practiced when doing this exercise.  Shadow boxing is actually a rehearsal of what you plan to do to your opponent when they are in the cage or ring with you.  Push the envelope as much as possible.  In other words, push yourself so that your pace and power are superior to any of your opponents.

### Shadow boxing with or without an opponent

When **shadow boxing**, work hard and fast while maintaining power and control.  Practice dictating the pace and knowing exactly where your punches are going.  Utilize your entire arsenal of defensive combinations, counters, and offensive combinations.  Use hand speed, power punching, hitting up and down, in and out, feinting, and above all, practice your positioning and breathing.

When working with an opponent be sure to keep at arms length.  If you start to move in or you find your opponent moving in, always continue to punch in front of their gloves.  This way you will be practicing your long-medium and medium-short range punches.

## Mirror Work

### Introduction

As in shadow boxing, the mirror is used to emulate your opponent and assist you in knowing exactly where you are punching.  Practice utilizing all of your weapons on the person in the mirror as if he or she is your enemy.  Work hard and fast, with power and control.  Dictate the pace, always knowing exactly where your punches are going.  Utilize your entire arsenal of defensive combinations, counters, offensive combinations, hand speed, power punching, hitting up, down, in, and out, feinting, and above all, your positioning and breathing.

**Look at yourself in the mirror as if you are the opponent**.  Punch at the chin, soft parts of the body, and the other body parts previously mentioned that serve to breakdown an opponent.  **Mirror work is just like shadow boxing** except that you are challenging yourself!

**Practice Stalking** (offensive and defensive positioning) when moving towards the mirror and practice your footwork and head movement when moving back and away from the mirror. Include some pivots, fakes, and feints. Always include the countering while practicing your defensive combinations. Make sure to throw your punches in bunches!

When practicing by your self use the **Defensive Drill** of placing a piece of tape about the width of a fist by 12 inches long, placing the bottom of the tape at chin level on the mirror. Your head and body should be placed directly in the middle of the tape. Practice the slip to the outside of the tape. You should be able to see your whole head (face) in the mirror. Now slip your head to the other side. Practice your bobbing and weaving making sure you are going under the lower end of the tape. Again, you should be able to see your whole head when you come up. Practice the blocking exercise, then the footwork.
See figure CV-57

Now start mixing them up getting different **combinations** going such as slipping and stepping, bobbing and stepping etc. You want to develop muscle memory as well.

Once you feel comfortable with your movements, begin **countering** to the head and body after every move. Practice, practice, and more practice is what it will take to perfect the defense and countering necessary to become a champion.
See figure CV-58

Start slow and easy obtaining correct positions. Once comfortable with the movement; start adding in the countering. Again, start slow and easy; getting the muscle memory down. After a while get mean, move and hit fast and hard, using power and control, and knowing where you are hitting at all times!

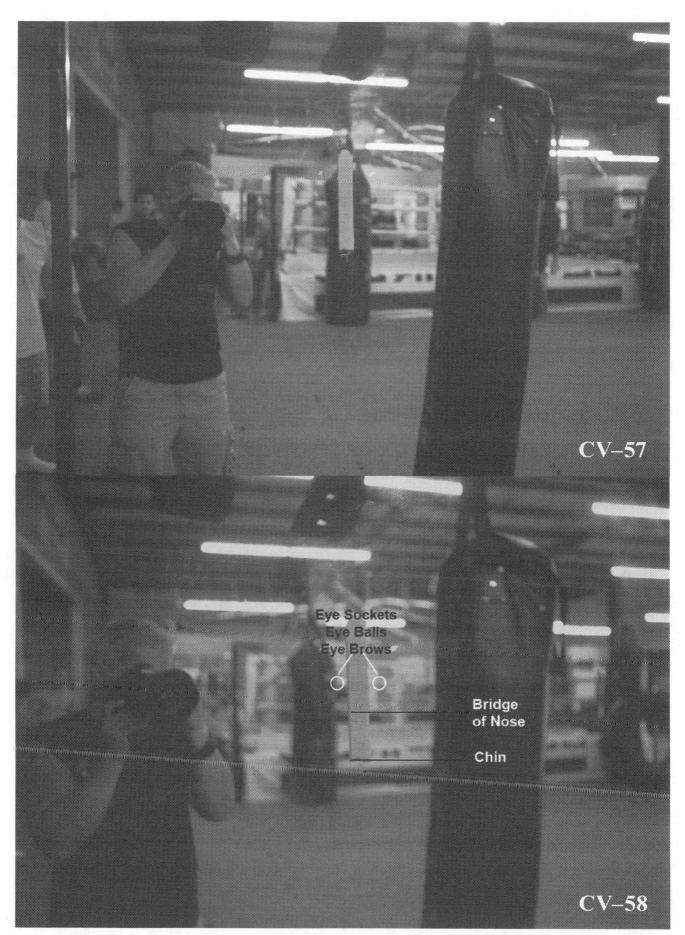

CV–57

Eye Sockets
Eye Balls
Eye Brows

Bridge
of Nose

Chin

CV–58

# NOTES

# VI BAG DRILLS

## Introduction

**Bag Drills** utilize a variety of bag types; punching bags, mitts, 2-end bags, speed bag, and the wall bag. All the varieties enable you to practice multiple skills while preparing for battle. If used correctly the bag drills will assist in making you a better champion fighter and a longer reigning champion as well.

## Punching Bag

There are normally 3-types of bags to beat on. Be sure to treat the bag like it is an opponent. Never lay on the bag with your head or stand in front of it since you would never work that way with an opponent. **Utilize your punching positions and combinations both defensively and offensively** to get more out of the bag than just beating on it. Size it up to your body. Hit at the chin, nose, and stomach level.
See figures CVI-1 thru CVI-3

- **The heavy bag** is for hard and heavy punching. Practice your favorite punch or punches along with as many offensive and defensive combinations as you can come up with. Work on hitting and moving side to side or taking one step back and then moving back in to deliver more punishment. Hit combinations and stay inside in-fighting or hit combinations and jab out to create another offensive position. Remember to double or triple up on punches, utilizing throwing punches in bunches! This bag is great for heavy weights.

- **The medium bag** is a nice combination of the light and heavy bag and will be utilized the same way as for the heavy and light bag. The medium bag is better for middle weight fighters.

- **The fast light bag** is for practicing your fast controlled punches and foot movement. You want to work to keep the light bag centered and controlled at times, not letting it fly all over the place. In other words, hit with power and control bringing your hands and arms back into position after each punch. Other times, use the constant movement of the bag to practice your footwork and upper body movement. Don't let the bag touch you. Use your footwork to maneuver side to side and in and out, never letting the bag hit you.

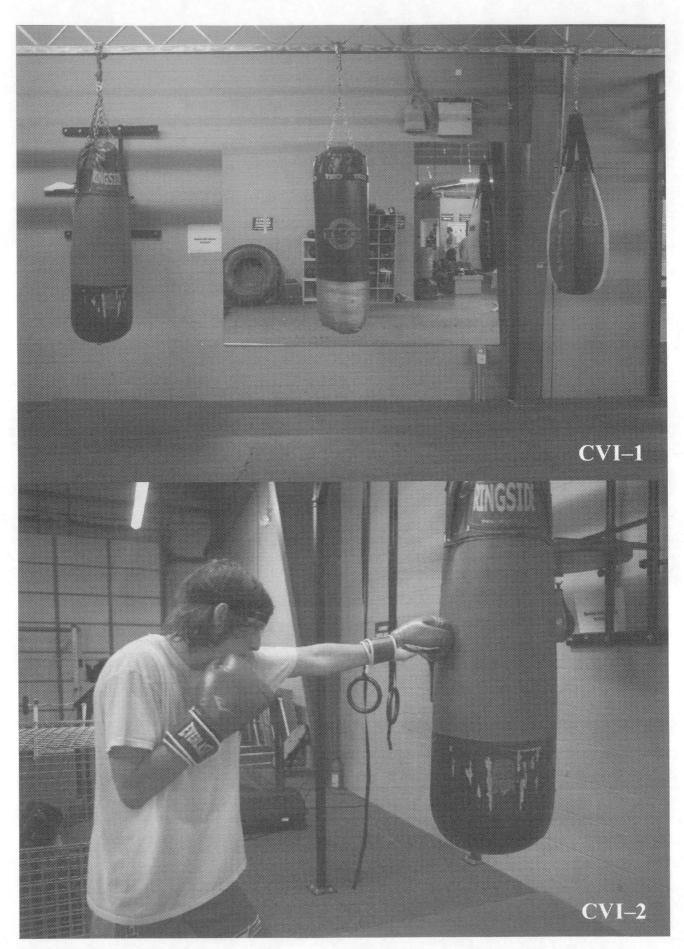

CVI–1

CVI–2

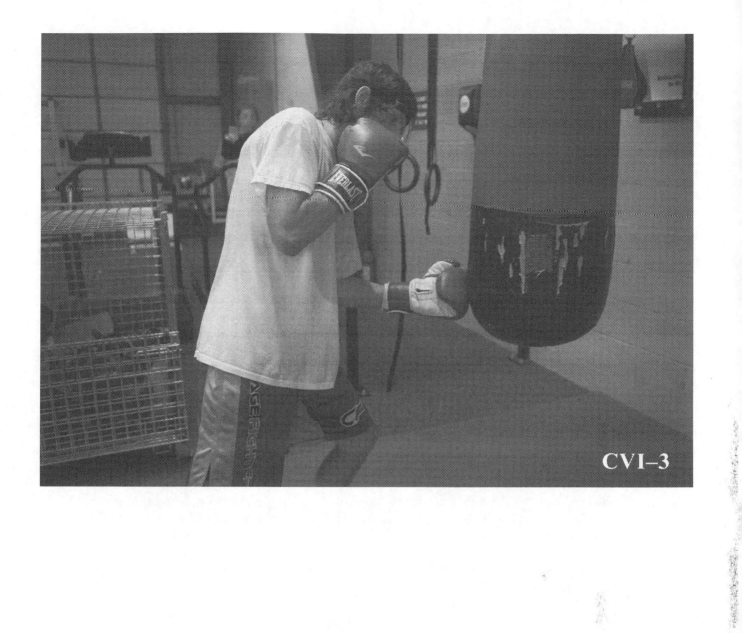

CVI–3

## Mitts

Both fighters will get something out of practicing the mitt work.
See figure CVI-4

- The fighter holding the mitts (**the holder**) will hold them in the correct boxing arm position practicing their (catching) blocking both soft and hard style. The holder practices their defensive moves while placing the mitts in strategic positions for the puncher. The mitt holder can also practice defensive movement by allowing the puncher get into their power positions and punch at the target with power and control. The holder must be able to hold the mitts firmly not letting the mitts come back and hit them. The holder can also throw punches at the puncher having them counter to the body or mitt.

- The **puncher** will be practicing their defensive moves, punching the mitts with power and control using continuous movement. Catch the holder moving in with quick fast punches and/or hard punishing strikes. Practice perfecting your favorite punch and then practice other punches like the 7-jabs, body shots, uppercuts, hooks, and combinations of these.

## 2-end bag

- Gauge your **distance** by putting your fully extended arm up (without locking the elbow) at the center of the ball. Hit the ball and move around, stop and check your position making sure you are the same distance from the bag as when you started.
See figure CVI-5

- Throw plenty of jabs plus **offensive and defensive combinations**. Practice the head and body movement while continuing to hit the bag. Begin punching using the long-medium position on the bag. Next, take the ½ step in and practice the medium-short range punching without getting hit by the bag.

- This exercise is good for your hand/eye coordination, your positioning, and building up your stamina.

## Speed Bag

- **Position** your elbows in while constantly hitting the bag. This assists in building up your muscle memory and arms to enable you to continue for a full round each and every time. Change up the speed, power, and striking styles.
See figures CVI-6 & CVI-7

- This exercise is also excellent for building up your stamina as well as hand/eye coordination.

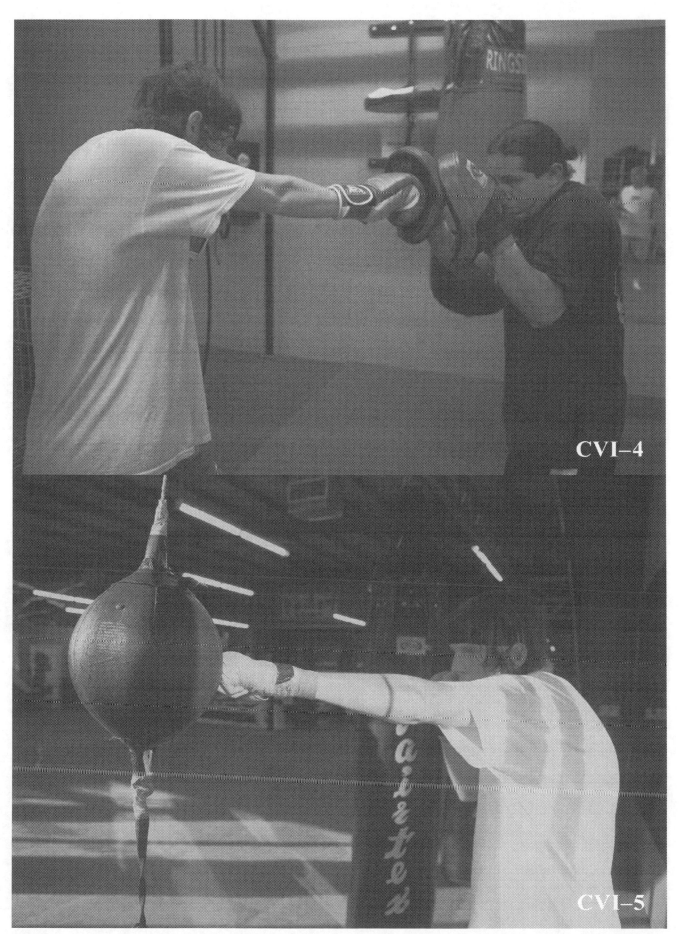

CVI–4

CVI–5

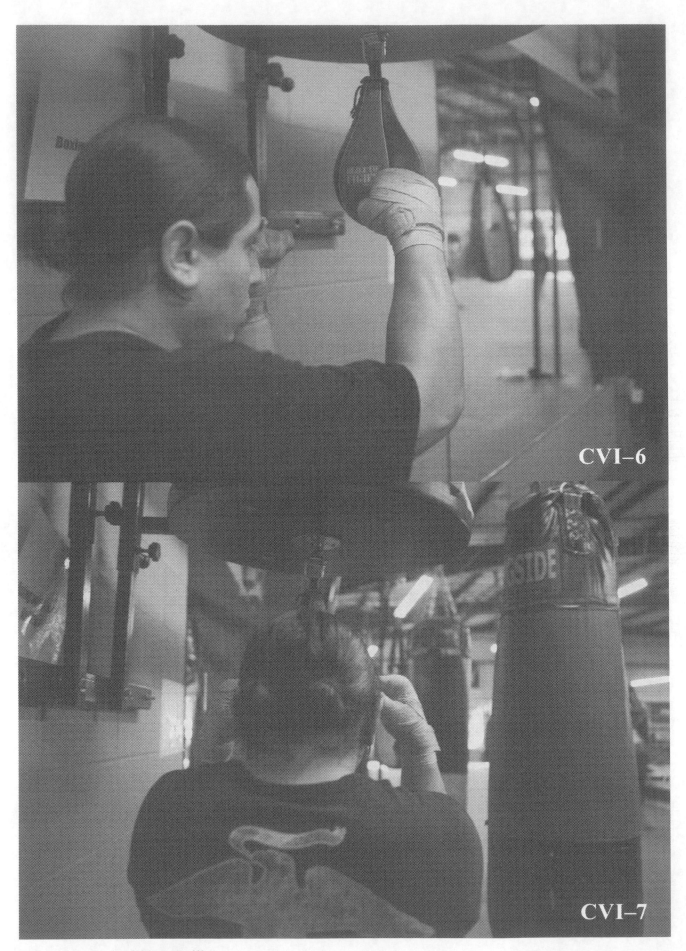

CVI–6

CVI–7

## The Wall Bag

Begin by **positioning** your body in the long-medium range. Then half step into the medium-close range.

See figures CVI-8 thru CVI-11

Practice all the defensive moves (slipping, bobbing, blocking, and footwork), countering on the bag while constantly moving. Hit exactly where you want to, using good solid punches as if the wall bag stole your woman (or man).

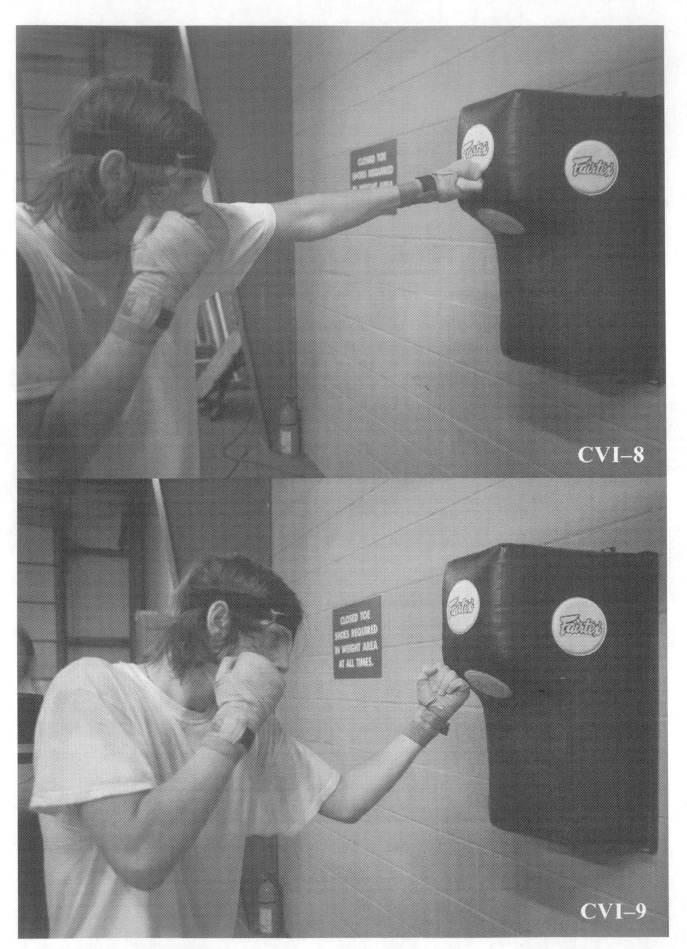

CVI–8

CVI–9

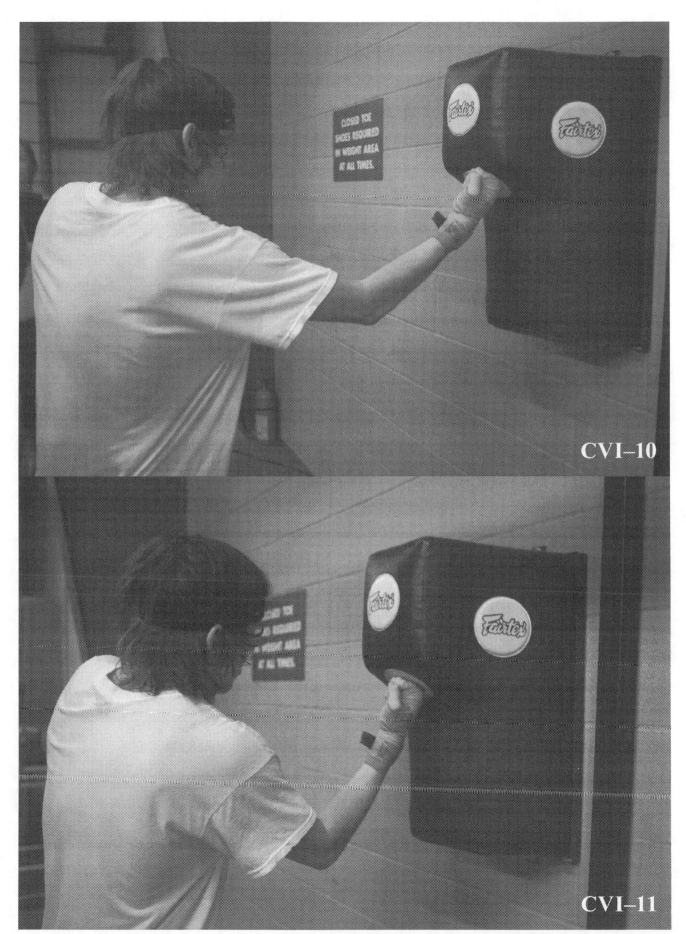

CVI–10

CVI–11

# NOTES

# VII SPARRING, FIGHT DAY, & CONCLUSION

## Sparring

## Introduction

The purpose of **sparring** is to practice and perfect all that you have been taught in the previous sections. Start off sparring at a 50-75% speed and power range. You must incorporate jabs, hooks, uppercuts, feints, body shots, and breathing into your sparring. If something doesn't work on one sparring partner, it does not mean it will not work on another.

Do not hesitate to try different combinations both offensively and defensively. If you practice everything you've been working on in the previous exercises your skills can only improve. You can and will eventually come up with combinations and moves that better suit your own style. You will also be able to adjust your style for each opponent during or in between rounds.

The body and head are not accustomed to being beat on, so in the beginning you will blink your eyes, feel nervous, your breathing will be erratic, and you might even get hurt by the punches. That's OK; it's all a part of the sparring. If your body is not ready for full contact; it will take a few sparring sessions to get it prepared for battle. Your head will have to build up its resistance to the punch through building up its bone mass. Your body will get tougher as you continue to spar. Your body and head will get used to the contact as you practice the various defenses and offenses.

Now that you've accomplished the hardest part of sparring, being hit, it is time to start picking up the pace. It's your turn to make the other person feel the pain.

Control your breathing and the pace while stalking your opponent, hitting hard with power and control. Know where you are hitting and most importantly, achieve the goal of winning every round. Sparring enhances the body, mind, and spirit of boxing.

- Your **sparring equipment** should consist of; a form fitted mouth piece, a headgear, 16oz sparring gloves (minimum), handwraps, and in some cases a cup. Most strikers do not use cups when sparring, all boxers do.
See figure CVII-1

- Your **sparring drills** should consist of mentally and physically practicing all that you've been taught. In the beginning you will find yourself first thinking and then doing. Then doing and thinking. Then just doing it. Your reflexes and movement; both defensively and offensively will fall into place. The eventual goal is to methodically take your sparring partner apart, each and every round. Again, when you first start sparring, remember to start at 50-75%. After a while you will be able to spar harder and faster with power and control at 100%. You should work with sparring partners that are more experienced than you and that know how to work. This will help you continue to improve.

When **sparring,** practice what you have been working on that week. Don't be afraid to get hit, it happens and is inevitable. Therefore, it is important to move on and learn from it. Practice everything that you've learned and perfect it during your sparring sessions.

**These are useful hints in sparring:**

- Keep your eyes wide open and on your opponent

- Control your breathing

- Watch every movement of your opponent

- Keep your mouth as firmly closed as possible

- Breathe through your nose

- Don't hold your muscles too tensely. If too stiff, you'll fatigue faster and impede your workout. Furthermore, you can't get the proper workout of stiff muscles

- Keep your movement controlled and stable

- Stay on the balls of your feet for quick movement

- Don't leap when practicing footwork

- Practice your long-mid range and mid-close range positioning

- Practice your in-fighting, on or off the cage or ropes

- Hit with the knuckles, don't slap!

- Know where you are hitting, aiming for those weak spots

- Do nothing in your sparring that you would not do in competition

- Take your sparring seriously, win every round

- Never lead blindly, and avoid hitting wildly

- Don't blink when you see your opponent's blow coming. Instead make a quick decision on your defense or offence

- Practice your defensive and offensive combinations

- Make your opponent miss and make them pay with counters

- Keep your chin and ass down, maintaining a solid foundation

- Be set to take a punch and give a punch

- Do not think about what kind of punch your opponent might throw. That will stop you from executing your own punches. In other words, be aware of them just don't dwell on them

- Fight your own style, don't let your opponent dictate the style that he wants you to use

- Have fun!

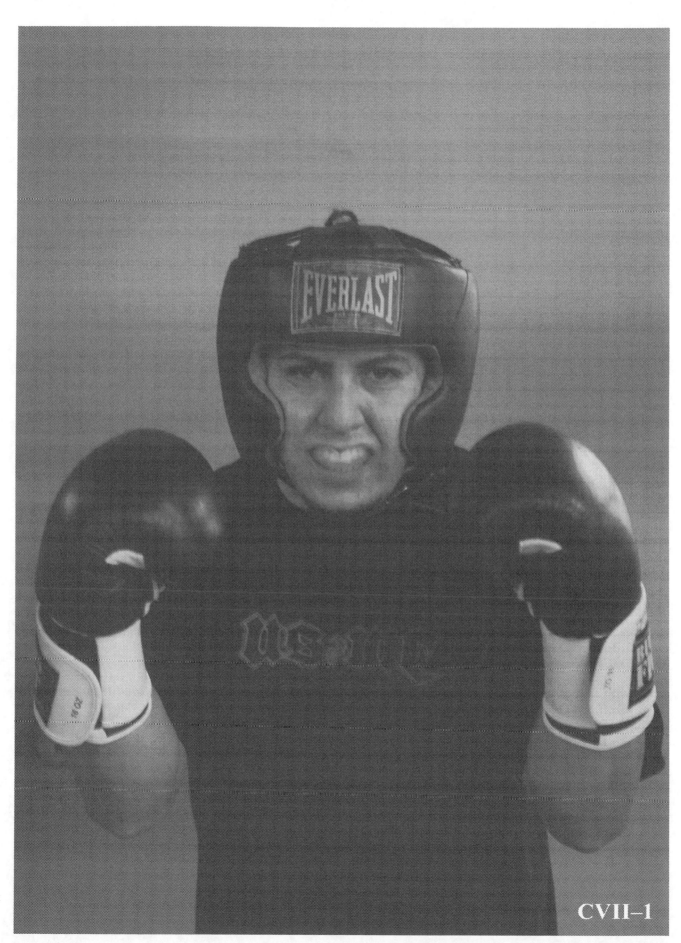

CVII–1

# NOTES

# FIGHT DAY

## Introduction

While relaxing there will be times when your heart will start racing and you might feel a little bit of anxiety. That's OK! This is where you practice the breathing exercise mentioned earlier. It's all a part of the lifestyle you have chosen when you decided to become an MMA Fighter. Deal with it and become what it is that you believe you are inside, and not what anybody else thinks, whether good or bad. You must believe that this is what you are and this is what you want to do.

With all the training you have been through you must believe that it is for your own personal reasons and that you want to be a champion. You are not training to be a chump for the other guy to beat on towards their way to the championship that is yours for the taking. You will achieve this by way of beating your opponent down and out, until the referee stops the bout, or you get tired, and **you don't get tired!**

**Control your breathing all day**. It is imperative to keep your heart rate at a smooth and calm pulse. If your heart is beating fast all day you might as well be running, thereby lowering your endurance, **so control it!**

## Pre-fight Study

Whenever possible, view your opponents past fights, studying them by yourself and/or with other people. Shadow box in front of the TV screen as if you are their opponent. Know your opponents strengths and weaknesses. This enables you to capitalize on your strengths!

The last two weeks before the fight should be as follows:

In **week two** you should be sharpening up your offensive and defensive moves. Test your conditioning to the maximum, pushing the envelope while getting your body, mind, and spirit into winning form.

During the **last week (Week One)** you should already be in great shape mentally, physically, and spiritually. You should be eating, sleeping and with the exercises you've been completing be ready for whatever comes at you. There will be times when an opponent is changed before the actual event. That's OK; you will only adjust your style as necessary. This should not bother you in the least, since you are the better fighter. You have been training harder, you are more skilled, and you have the mental strength to beat anyone that comes at you attempting to hurt and defeat you.

Never try to radically change your own boxing style or add new moves the week before a bout. It will confuse you and may cause you to return to think and do rather than, just doing it!

## Attitude:

If you want to be successful, remember to be civil in and out of the ring. Be respectful of your opponent whenever possible. You are both MMA fighters looking to win the crowd in order to be a great fighter, champion, and person. Do not act ignorant towards the crowd, your opponent, the referee, or even your cornermen. Show some class in and out of the ring or cage and the public will love you. That, my friend, is how true champions are proudly remembered.

## Conclusion

This guide covers a lot of material in a small package. You may not use all the materials or weapons given to you in this guide book but what you do use will assist you in getting the best out of yourself and your training partner. Utilizing these techniques will keep you in the fight game longer than not using them at all.

There's an old saying handed down to me from my boxing coach (Jerry) back in the day, it goes:

*He who hits and moves away will live to hit another day...*
*He who hits and moves in will score a quick win...*

Which one will you do?

*This is the first edition. The next edition will cover strength exercises, conditioning, combinations, elbows, plus exercises related to positioning for body shots and backhands. Listening, watching the other corner between rounds. Including the California Amateur Mixed Martial Arts Organization (CAMO) guidelines.*

To contact the author e-mail: mmastrikersguide@gmail.com

Printed in the United States
by Baker & Taylor Publisher Services